14-Day Detox

FOR WEIGHT LOSS

14-Day Detox

FOR WEIGHT LOSS

A Meal Plan
& Easy Recipes
to Lose Weight, Fast

KIM McDEVITT, MPH, RD

PHOTOGRAPHY BY HÉLÈNE DUJARDIN

ROCKRIDGE PRESS

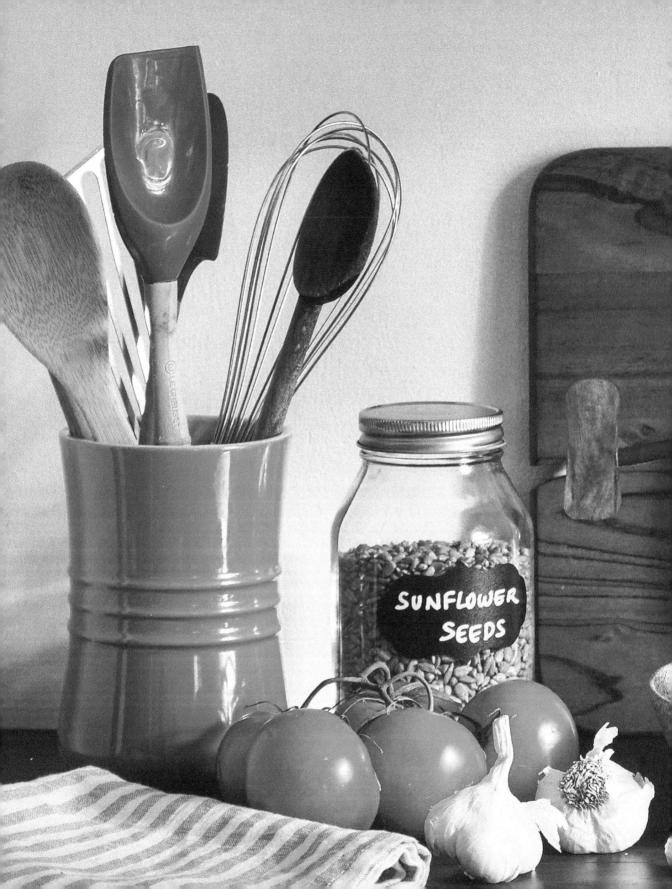

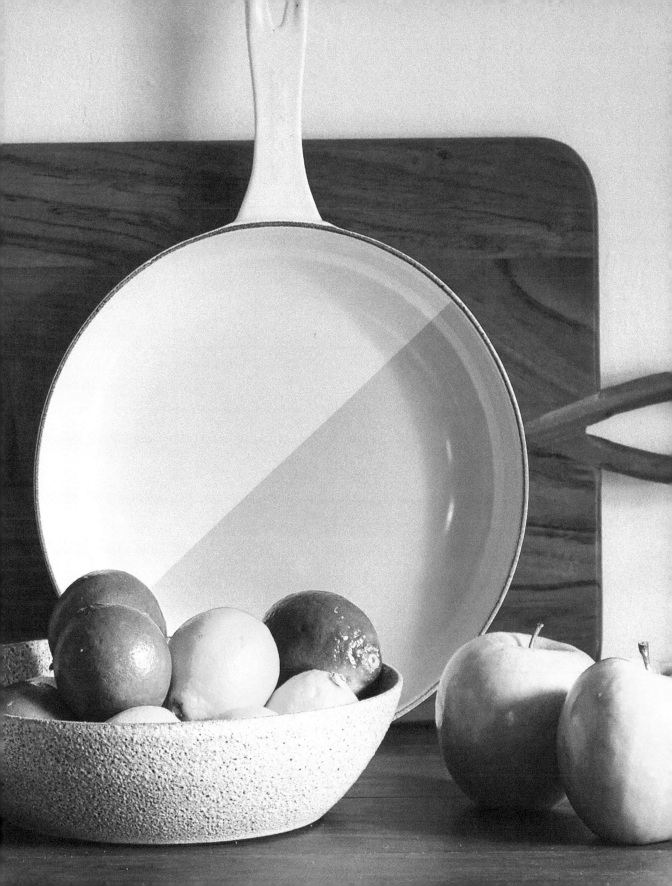

For general information on our other products and services or to obtain technical support, please contact our Customer Care Department within the United States at (866) 744-2665, or outside the United States at (510) 253-0500.

Rockridge Press publishes its books in a variety of electronic and print formats. Some content that appears in print may not be available in electronic books, and vice versa.

TRADEMARKS: Rockridge Press and the Rockridge Press logo are trademarks or registered trademarks of Callisto Media Inc. and/or its affiliates, in the United States and other countries, and may not be used without written permission. All other trademarks are the property of their respective owners. Rockridge Press is not associated with any product or vendor mentioned in this book.

Interior and Cover Designer: Richard Tapp
Photo Art Director/Art Manager: Sara Feinstein
Editor: Cecily McAndrews
Production Editor: Ashley Polikoff
Photography: Hélène Dujardin
Photography © 2020 Hélène Dujardin.
Food styling by Anna Hampton

ISBN: Print 978-1-64611-676-8
eBook 978-1-64611-677-5

R0

To my husband, John, who pushed me to chase my dreams of becoming a wellness expert, who believed in me long before I believed in myself, and without whom this beautiful life of mine wouldn't exist.

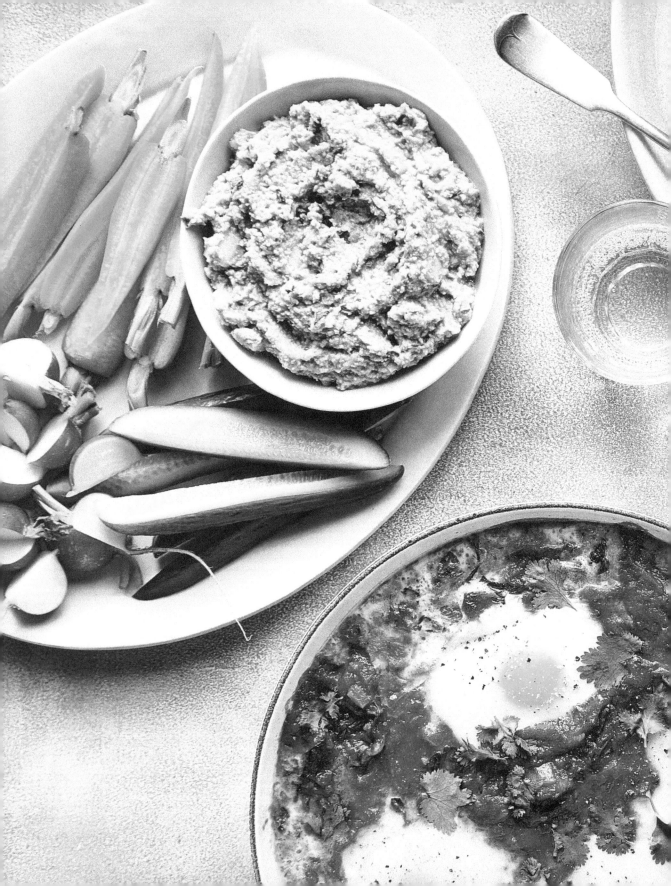

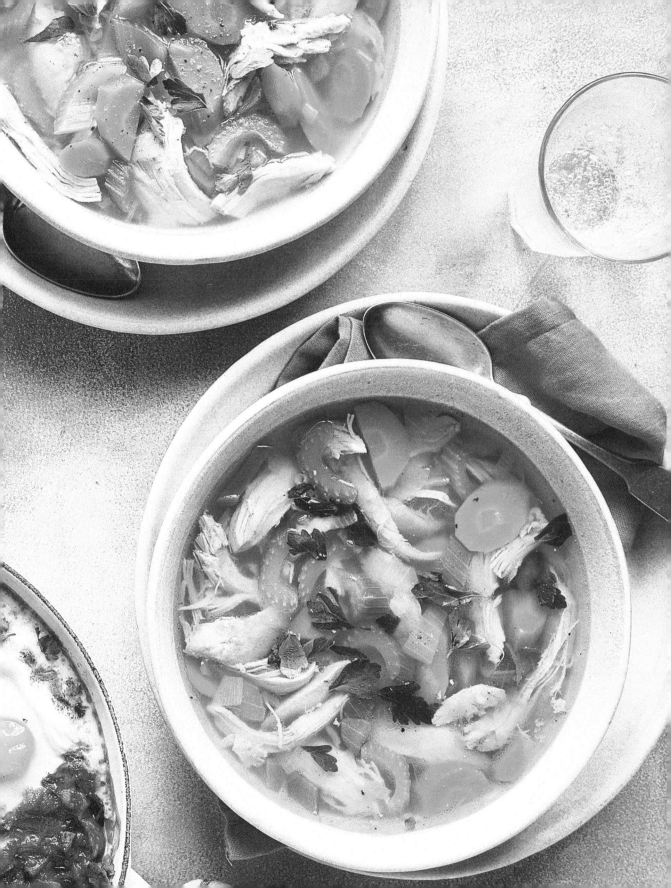

contents

introduction

Congratulations! If you're reading this, that means you've decided to embark on, or are considering embarking on, an exciting journey over the next 14 days. That is a big step, and one that is worth celebrating.

This book presents you with a two-week starting plan, but it also provides the recipes that will enable you to keep going after you've completed the starting plan. The book will also teach you how to make food choices that will enhance your general well-being. At the same time, it will educate you on, and give you the confidence to make, good food choices that you can take with you beyond the 14 days.

So, who am I and why am I the right person to help you get there? For nearly my entire adult life, I've been fascinated by nutrition and how our food choices support our health. So fascinated, in fact, that I left a career in marketing to pursue a masters in public health (with a focus on human nutrition) and became a registered dietitian. My goal then, and now, is to help people navigate the overwhelming number of food choices, fad diets, and products lining grocery store shelves. Through my education and experience, I've been able to teach people that food can either lift you up or drag you down, both physically and mentally. With this understanding, people can start to connect what they eat with how they feel.

My approach is simple: Limit refined and processed foods and shift your choices to include whole foods and better-for-you options. Replace overprocessed choices devoid of nutrition with nourishing, satisfying meals and snacks.

With this in mind, I'll help you create your own personal eating plan that supports both your taste buds and your health.

My hope is that this plan will allow you to walk away from the next 14 days feeling physically and mentally lighter; that you'll notice increased energy levels, improved mental clarity, and, yes, weight loss; that you'll feel empowered to keep pursuing or maintaining your goals; and that you'll start reaching for nutrient-dense whole foods over highly processed alternatives because you know that these options are satisfying and make you *feel* better.

As we grow and evolve, our diet should grow and evolve with us. This detox plan and the recipes in this book can help you be a bit more intentional when it comes to your diet's evolution. With a little thought and effort, and by specifically focusing on foods that will support positive changes in your diet, you will ultimately improve your overall well-being. And who wouldn't want that?

Detox Fundamentals

Let's begin your 14-day detox with a strong foundation. I'm going to walk you through why a detox is a good idea, and how to make this detox work for you. I'm also going to highlight foods to eat and foods to avoid, which will guide your grocery shopping and eating habits for the next two weeks, and provide the ingredients for a delicious, deprivation-free detox.

Defining Detox

The term "detox" may seem intense. You may associate it with hunger, hard work, or boring foods. This book is going to help you take some simple steps to shift that mind-set. Instead, consider this detox to be a simple reset of your system, one that can be enjoyable and achievable. Consider it to be a gain, not a loss. You'll be able to spend the next 14 days developing a better version of yourself by embracing the foods that support your health and energy and limiting the foods that drag you down.

This detox isn't meant to be a test of will. It's easy to follow, and easy to follow through. Committing to this detox doesn't mean you won't ever be able to enjoy your favorite sweet treat again. But it does mean that for the next 14 days you'll focus on preparing and eating foods that are clean, healthy, and nutrient-dense. And, if you stick to this plan, you'll start seeing all sorts of results. You'll notice that your pants will start to feel looser. You'll start feeling more energized. You'll even find yourself sleeping more soundly. And with all of these positives, you'll start to enjoy, and even crave, the healthy meals so much that you'll begin to form new eating habits.

Why 14 Days?

I focus on 14 days because it is such a manageable chunk of time. At the same time, two weeks is long enough to allow you to see progress toward your goals.

This detox centers mostly on the numerous healthy food options you can have, but there are still some off-limits foods. Some of the foods you'll avoid for the 14 days, you can begin to include again after the two weeks are up. Others, I am hopeful that you'll continue to limit even after the detox period ends. After the two weeks, I believe that the changes you'll see in yourself will inspire you to carry most of this plan into your everyday life for a long time to come, while still feeling as though you can enjoy a glass of wine every now and again or share some fries with your family when you're out to dinner.

How to Use This Book

In the following pages, you'll find guidance on preparing for your detox, a day-by-day meal plan, all the recipes you need to pull it off, and some helpful tips to make nutritious and healthy food choices in the long term, beyond the 14 days of the detox. Of course, you don't have to be in the midst of the detox to enjoy the nutritious and delicious meals you'll find in this book, so feel free to skip right to the recipes, starting on page 37.

The recipes in the book are meant to be flexible. There isn't a one-size-fits-all path to better health and we're realistic about what makes a successful detox. Explore the recipes in this book and get creative. Swap recipes in the meal plan for ones that suit your tastes better, or switch up ingredients to make them work for you and your family. Remember, it's about progress, not perfection.

This detox should work *for* you. You won't need to spend 18 hours in the kitchen each day over the next two weeks, cooking extensive meals with unique ingredients. These meals contain ingredients that are familiar and easy to find at the grocery store. Nearly all the recipes you'll find within this book will come together in 30 minutes or less (especially when you've done some prep work ahead of time), and have fewer than 10 ingredients. And as a bonus, nearly every recipe is designed to have leftovers for an easy lunch or for when you don't feel like cooking another dinner.

Keep in mind that whether you start seeing positive changes right away and drop a few pounds in the first few days, or don't see the scale nudge for the first week, it's okay! Everyone's body will respond differently and at a different pace to these new habits. Try not to get frustrated; just stick with it. Losing weight might be your primary goal but there are so many more benefits that you'll gain from reducing your processed food, carb, sugar, and unhealthy fat intake.

That said, you should definitely consult with your doctor before engaging in any new diet or weight loss regimen. Odds are, your doctor will be excited that you're focusing on making nutritious choices with your food. But you should make sure that the plan that this book outlines is a healthy option for you based on your medical history and any other specific restrictions you might have.

Foods to Enjoy on Your Detox

As you go through the next two weeks, you should focus on the fact that there are so many foods you CAN eat. Don't focus on the foods that are off-limits. While sticking to these foods will be an adjustment, the plan will get you closer to feeling like the best version of yourself.

Vegetables

Vegetables are packed with nutrients like vitamins, minerals, and fiber. They help fight inflammation, aid in digestion, and maintain blood sugar levels. In most cases, you have the go-ahead to eat vegetables in unlimited quantities.

LEAFY GREENS

Leafy greens include basic salad greens like baby spinach and arugula, but also kale, Swiss chard, bok choy, and others. These greens are rich in vitamins, low in calories, and should make an appearance at nearly every meal.

CRUCIFEROUS VEGETABLES

High in fiber, these veggies include Brussels sprouts, broccoli, cauliflower, and cabbage. These vegetables take on different, delicious flavors depending on how they are prepared. Add them to at least one meal every day. Bonus: You can eat this group of vegetables with abandon!

Fruits

A lot of diets caution you not to eat fruits because of their higher sugar content. However, fruit sugars are naturally occurring, easily digested, and can be a great source of energy. Fruit is also high in vitamins and minerals, antioxidants, phytochemicals, and fiber. Plus, when you're omitting lots of processed foods with added sugars, a sweet, juicy piece of fruit can feel like a treat.

Still, you need to choose your fruits wisely, as some fruits are better than others during the first part of this journey. Lower-glycemic fruits (meaning those that raise your blood sugar more slowly) such as berries, apples, pears, and citrus, are better choices.

Protein

Protein is one of the three macronutrients that make up food (carbohydrates and fats are the others). Protein breaks down into amino acids, which your body needs but cannot make itself. Protein comes from both plant and animal sources and this detox plan has both. If you are a vegetarian, you will find recipes that include eggs. There are also a handful of vegan recipes in here. Vegetarians and vegans may need to boost meals with protein from sources such as hemp seeds, beans, or vegan protein powder.

Our cells rely on protein for structure, function, and regulation of body tissues and organs. Protein helps repair body tissues, maintain muscle mass, and regulate hormones. It also keeps blood sugar and energy levels more stable, which helps reduce carbohydrate cravings.

MEAT

If choosing only certain products to buy organic, meat is the first I would choose. Grass-fed beef is one of the best options, but buying organic or even antibiotic- and hormone-free is better than conventional. Beyond the quality of the meat, the cut matters, as you should be mindful of saturated fats. Reach for leaner cuts, such as pork tenderloin, trimmed pork loin chops, flank steak, ground bison, or 90% or leaner ground beef and lamb.

POULTRY

Always look for organic or antibiotic-free poultry. Chicken and turkey breasts, backs, and legs are great options for roasting. Other good choices are organic chicken sausages, ground turkey, and nitrate-free turkey from the deli. I also love grabbing a prepared rotisserie chicken when I'm short on time.

EGGS

Eggs make a versatile and delicious protein option. While the bulk of the protein is found in the whites, don't shy away from eating one or two yolks each day. The yolk contains all the egg's beneficial fat-soluble vitamins (A, D, E, K), calcium, iron, B vitamins, and choline, as well as powerful antioxidants. If possible, purchase pasture-raised or organic.

SEAFOOD

Fish is an amazing lean protein source that may also deliver a boost of omega-3 healthy fats. Choose wild-caught or sustainably farmed fish, which will have the most nutrients. To

be certain, you can download an app to help guide your choice, such as the one offered by the Monterey Bay Aquarium. My top recommendations are salmon, shrimp, scallops, and cod or haddock. Canned fish, including salmon, tuna, and sardines, are also great choices.

SOY

Soy can be controversial, but I believe it is a fine choice when consumed in moderation and not in isolate forms (like powdered soy protein isolate, which is frequently found in packed snack foods). I like tofu, edamame, and tempeh for a plant-based protein addition to any meal.

Healthy Fats

Fats are referred to by many names. They are often grouped together as either "good fats" or "bad fats." Good fats (also known as are known as mono- or polyunsaturated fats) are the ones to choose, especially over the next 14 days. Sources include raw nuts and seeds, fatty fish, avocados and avocado oil, and olive oil, and you'll work to incorporate these into your daily diet in controlled portions. Aside from tasting great, they provide a boost of energy, help you feel full, and allow your body to absorb fat-soluble vitamins. We'll discuss bad fats a little later.

Some of the most important fats for your diet are omega-3 fatty acids. They are a type of polyunsaturated fat found in popular foods like salmon and flax. This diet staple reduces inflammation, boosts muscle performance, and improves cell function.

Better Beverages

Nothing is better than water. Water is critical for nearly every single one of our body's functions and you'll want to prioritize it over the next 14 days. Staying hydrated is key to losing weight. The general rule is to drink at least half your body weight in ounces every day: Take the number of pounds, divide that in half, and that is the number of fluid ounces you should be drinking. I love adding some flavor to my water with mint leaves or sliced cucumber, lemon, or orange slices.

In addition to water, unsweetened tea or flavored seltzer can be good choices. But be a label sleuth, as many ready-to-drink teas are sweetened, either with sugar or sugar substitutes, or have other undesirable additives.

Salt and Seasonings

Adding spices, herbs, and salt is one of the best ways to add flavor to a meal without calories. Fresh herbs, such as basil, parsley, and cilantro, and spices like cinnamon will really bring meals to

SHOULD I BUY ORGANIC?

When we think of organic, we typically think first of fruits and vegetables. But the term organic applies to foods all over the grocery store, including packaged foods, dairy, meats, and eggs. Organic is the best option you can buy because the label indicates that a product has not been grown or raised with 700+ possible different chemicals out there. Of course, you do pay a premium for certified organic goods.

Still, there are many ways to enjoy the benefits of organic foods without the price tag. Look for locally grown produce, which is oftentimes organic, but is not officially certified. Buy fruits and vegetables that are in season, which often helps reduce cost. Buy on-sale or store-brand organic (which is just as good and usually less costly). Overall, I always urge people to buy the best-quality food that will fit in their budget, so use this as your guide.

life. Condiments also fit here, because many of them are low in calories but high in flavor. Some top choices to start using include apple cider vinegar, Dijon mustard, lemon juice, and tamari (gluten-free soy sauce).

Foods to Limit

Limiting a food doesn't necessarily mean cutting it out of your diet entirely or forever. But for the next two weeks, these are foods that you'll want to eat sparingly and in small portions. There's room for these foods in a healthy diet, but these two weeks are about cleansing your palate and starting fresh; too much of these items works against that goal.

Starchy Vegetables

Starchy vegetables include carrots, beets, winter squash, potatoes, and sweet potatoes. Despite including fiber, antioxidants, and essential vitamins, these vegetables also have a higher sugar and starch content and should therefore be eaten in moderation. So, although they roast wonderfully and can be healthy, when looking to lose weight, it's very important to be mindful of portion sizes.

Legumes

Legumes include beans, chickpeas, lentils, and peanuts. Beans and lentils offer the body a combination of fiber, protein, and carbohydrate all in one. That said, because they are a higher-carbohydrate protein option and can be difficult for the body to digest at times, it is important to watch your portions over the next 14 days.

Grains

When it comes to weight loss, you should limit grains. When eaten in proper portions, and not as the focus of a meal, they can be a healthy food to include, but limiting them is key.

In fact, for the first 7 days of your detox, I'll likely suggest you omit them almost entirely, starting to slowly add them back during week 2. Why? Grains can be difficult for the body to digest. And because they are a concentrated carbohydrate, which is converted to sugar in the body, they are also quickly stored as fat when eaten in excess (which is easy to do), show up as water weight, and sometimes result in bloat, brain fog, and cravings.

That said, whole grains do give your body fiber and sometimes even a bit of protein.

I'll guide you on how and when to use grains, so by the end of the 14 days you'll be confident about when to incorporate them and when to skip.

Nuts and Seeds

Nuts and seeds offer your body not only healthy fats, but protein and fiber as well. Because they are high in calories, eat only a small handful at a time.

Saturated Fats

Not all fats are created equal, which is why they are included in all three categories: Foods to Enjoy, Foods to Limit, and Foods to Avoid. Fats deliver the most calories per gram of food (9 calories), more than protein or carbohydrates. This means that a smaller amount delivers a higher total calorie count, so portion size really counts.

Saturated fats, found in foods like red meat, full-fat dairy, coconut, and butter, have been associated with negative health effects, like an increased risk of heart disease. Limit saturated fats and only consume occasionally.

Caffeinated Beverages

Feel free to keep coffee as part of your morning routine, but try to limit yourself to 1 to 2 cups (which is around 200 milligrams of caffeine each day). Caffeine can be beneficial; it can increase stamina when you're working out and can help to speed up your metabolism. But excessive caffeine consumption can disrupt hunger cues and food cravings and can really alter your sleep patterns. Sleep is always really important, but especially so during your detox.

Foods to Avoid

Naturally there are going to be some foods we recommend cutting out entirely for the next 14 days and, arguably, forever. These off-limits foods are known to contribute to weight gain, cravings, inflammation, and even more severe health issues. If you do ultimately reintroduce these foods into your diet, you'll want to keep the mind-set that these should be an occasional food or treat.

Processed Foods

These days, processed and packaged foods are the norm; they're tempting in part because of convenience. But what makes them so bad? Often, they comprise some combination of refined grains, processed sugars, and bad-for-you fats. Put simply, processed grains and processed sugars make you gain weight. What's more, so many packaged snacks, dips, and salad dressings are full of additives and unnecessary ingredients, such as artificial flavors, colors, preservatives, and excess sodium. My rule is that if I don't understand every single ingredient listed on the box or bag, I try to find a better, "cleaner" option.

Note that a couple of the meals in the book include bacon, ham, and chicken sausage, which are technically "processed" meats. I've included them because they're fast, delicious options, and it's possible to find "clean" versions. Look for products that are nitrate-free, have no sugar added, and are from a brand that you trust, like Applegate, which uses all humanely raised, hormone- and antibiotic-free meat.

There are plenty of convenient options that aren't processed. Look for packaged foods free of anything artificial and convenience options like prechopped produce.

Refined Sugars

Sugar is hiding everywhere and it's arguably the most important ingredient to pay attention to when it comes to weight and health. It's in the obvious places, but also in sneaky spots like barbecue sauce, salad dressings, and tomato sauce. Even lunch meats can sometimes contain unnecessary added sugar. Sugar is a cheap way for producers to enhance flavor, but it lends non-nutritive calories that lead to overeating, cravings, unhealthy weight gain, blood sugar imbalance, diabetes, high blood pressure, bloating, and more. Avoiding this added sugar will help you sleep better, give you more energy, clear your skin, and contribute to healthy weight goals.

Gluten

Gluten is actually a protein that is found in wheat, barley, spelt, and rye. Those with a true intolerance (known as celiac disease) cannot digest gluten. Many of us have developed a gluten sensitivity, however, because it is so prevalent in our diets. Symptoms include digestive bloating or constipation, physical fatigue, acne, or headaches. It is best to avoid gluten in the 14-day detox and any clean-eating plan.

Dairy

There's a lot of confusion around whether you should eat dairy. For some, when eaten in moderation from high-quality sources, dairy can be a fine food choice. Others, however, may have a sensitivity that they don't even notice until they omit dairy completely. Deleting dairy may suddenly clear up allergies, acne, and/or poor digestion. Because so many people do have a dairy sensitivity, you'll cut out all forms of dairy for the next 14 days, including milk products, yogurt, cheese, and butter.

Unhealthy Fats

Otherwise known as the "bad fats" I mentioned earlier, this is a group of fats that you want to keep out of your diet. Trans fats are the worst offenders, as they are a cheap by-product of a commercial chemical process and are proven to raise the amount of harmful LDL cholesterol in your body while also reducing the good HDL cholesterol and contributing to inflammation. Stay clear of hydrogenated or partially hydrogenated vegetable oils, soybean oil, and margarine.

Soda

Study after study has connected health issues such as diabetes and weight gain to the high sugar content in regular soda, while diet sodas have been repeatedly linked to high-risk digestive disorders. Soda is filled with artificial colors, flavors, and additives that frankly have no place in our bodies.

And while I know on occasion it can feel like a delicious treat, your best bet is to cut it out except for on the very rarest of occasions—at least for the 14 days, and in a perfect world, forever.

Alcohol

There are plenty of okay reasons to enjoy an alcoholic beverage a few nights a week. But over the next 14 days, skip it. Alcohol is a perceived toxin to the body that can tax your system and disrupt your sleep. It also contains a lot of calories. Let your liver reset over the next two weeks and give it a rest from the alcohol.

DO I NEED A SUPPLEMENT?

Supplements are exactly what they sound like—a way to add to your existing diet. They should be used to fill in the gaps and support your health goals. Everyone could use a boost of omega-3 fatty acids and a probiotic. Those who eat a predominantly plant-based diet should consider B vitamins, and those of us who don't spend 10-plus months of the year outside in the sun should consider vitamin D. Collagen and protein powder can be nice complements to meals, because they help to keep you full and your blood sugar stable. Adding supplements is a personal choice and you should always consult your doctor first.

Purging Your Pantry

Get into the habit of cleaning out your pantry seasonally. Start by doing a cleaning before this detox. I tell my clients to resist one time at the store so that they don't have to resist an item repeatedly in their pantries!

Some pantry items can be set aside to reincorporate in moderation after the two weeks. But for the most part, get rid of that temptation. Purge all the processed foods, salty snacks, and sweet treats that are going to set you back. Now you have room for some better options. Check out the whole chart of swaps on the following page.

THE MANY NAMES OF SUGAR

Added sugar is everywhere, so become a sugar sleuth in order to eliminate as much of it as you can. Read nutrition labels and look for that "added sugar" line. The lower the number, the better. Check the ingredients list for these entries, which are just different names for sugar:

- Agave or agave nectar
- Brown sugar
- Cane sugar
- Carob syrup
- Coconut sugar
- Confectioners' (powdered) sugar
- Corn syrup
- Dextrose
- Evaporated cane syrup or juice
- Fructose
- Glucose
- High fructose corn syrup
- Honey
- Maple
- Molasses
- Sucrose
- Table sugar
- Turbinado sugar

UNHEALTHY PANTRY STAPLES	BETTER-FOR-YOU ADDITION
Bottled salad dressing with added sugar	Oils: extra-virgin olive oil, avocado oil, sesame oil Vinegars: apple cider vinegar, champagne vinegar, balsamic vinegar
Jarred pasta or pizza sauce with added sugar	Pasta sauce without added sugar Diced canned tomatoes
Quick-cooking grain kits (with flavor packets), such as rice pilaf and flavored instant oats	Quinoa, gluten-free rolled oats, wild rice, lentil or chickpea pasta
Canned beans, vegetables, or fruits with high sodium, added sugars, or added ingredients	Single-ingredient canned beans Unsweetened applesauce and pumpkin puree
Packaged sweet treats like cookies and candy	Dried fruits (with no added sugar or sulfites) 70 percent cacao dark chocolate Dark chocolate sweetened with stevia or monk fruit (like Lily's)
Roasted salted nuts	Raw or roasted unsalted nuts: almonds, walnuts, cashews, pistachios Seeds: ground flax, chia, sunflower, pumpkin
Sweeteners: granulated sugar, brown sugar, aspartame, sucralose	Organic cane sugar, coconut palm sugar, honey, molasses, monk fruit sweetener, organic liquid stevia
White flour	Blanched almond flour, coconut flour, oat flour, spelt flour

Cleaning Out Your Fridge and Freezer

You'll also want to do a deep clean of your refrigerator and freezer. Beyond staples, you'll find that each week you start with a full fridge and end with a nearly empty one. Why? Because you'll be filling it with predominantly fresh produce, proteins, and more.

Refrigerator

Purge items with poor-quality ingredients and exchange them for better ones. For instance, swap artificially flavored breakfast syrup for real maple syrup, bottled salad dressings for homemade, and flavored yogurts for plain ones. Poor-quality added sugars, like high fructose corn syrup, often make their way into ketchup and BBQ sauces, so be a label sleuth! Also, remove fruit juices or soda.

You'll be filling your fridge each week with delicious fresh produce and lean proteins. In addition to that, here are some staples that I always want on hand:

- Condiments: tamari, sriracha, Dijon mustard, organic low- or no-sugar added ketchup, avocado oil mayonnaise, pure maple syrup
- Pure lemon or lime juice, or lemons and limes
- Organic whole eggs, pure liquid eggs, and liquid egg whites (for ease of use)
- Unsweetened nondairy milk, such as almond, coconut, or oat
- Plain organic Greek yogurt (if and when you add dairy back into your diet, post-detox) or unsweetened or low-sugar (9 grams or less per serving) nondairy yogurts, such as almond, coconut, or oat
- Sparkling water

Freezer

Stock up! Give your future self the gift of an easy, healthy meal. You can easily stockpile high-quality meats when they go on sale, as well as wild-caught sustainable fish, frozen vegetables and fruits (just as nutritious and even easier than fresh), and leftover batches of tomato sauce, homemade soups, and more.

Here's a freezer list to get you started:

- Wild-caught seafood, including halibut, cod, shrimp, and salmon
- Grass-fed ground beef or turkey
- Organic chicken breasts
- Frozen vegetables: peas, broccoli, riced cauliflower, green beans
- Frozen fruit: all berries
- Bone broths and stocks

2

The Meal Plans
& Beyond

Now that you have a fundamental understanding of basic nutrition
principles, including which foods are good, better, and best for you,
let's put your new understanding into practice. In this chapter, you'll
find strategies, meal plans, and shopping lists to equip you with
the tools and confidence boost you need to launch your detox.

Detox Your Routine

There's a saying about developing new habits: "If nothing changes, then nothing changes." Which is simply a blithe way of expressing that you can't keep doing what you've been doing if you want to make a change in your life. No matter how you cut it, though, we are creatures of habit. We get into a fixed routine and, eventually, anything that falls outside of that routine feels uncomfortable and unnatural. And eating (the what, where, when, and how of it) becomes part of our comfortable routine.

But you're doing this detox to disrupt the routine, right? With that in mind, it's important to examine your daily routine and determine how some simple tweaks can support your goals for this detox diet. The most important routine disruption in the next two weeks will be to change the "what" part. We all have comfort foods that we look to when we need an emotional boost. For the next two weeks, commit to purging your diet of the foods that don't support your well-being or health.

You won't be able to completely overhaul every single part of your daily routine in the next two weeks, nor should you. And this means you're still going to be engaging in many of the same behaviors and facing many of the same emotions, whether it's watching TV at night or dealing with the stress of work. And if you have those salty or sweet treats tempting you from the back of the pantry, trust me, you're going to dig them out before the detox is over. But, if you've removed the temptation entirely, when you do reach for a snack to make it through a tough afternoon, it will be something that's on the detox-approved list. And, over the next two weeks, these nutritious and healthful snacks will start to become part of your new routine.

The Emotional Eating Worksheet

On the next page are some situations with which you may be able to identify. If you have a plan, you won't let yourself get into a situation that will derail all your good efforts. Remove temptation from your pantry, stock your fridge with smart choices, and always have a game plan to combat triggers and moments of weakness. Because when faced with temptation, the chances of you reaching for a trigger food are high, despite your best intentions.

THE SITUATION	TRIGGER FOOD	THE SUBSTITUTION
I wait too long or don't have time to eat breakfast	Anything fast and tempting when you're starving—bagel with cream cheese, muffin, donut, candy jar at work	Blues and Greens Smoothie (page 39) Fruity Yogurt Parfait (page 45) to go Hard-boiled eggs Piece of fruit
3 p.m. slump	Candy, sweet treats, salty snacks	Matcha Latte (page 62), Simple Homemade Hummus (page 53) with veggies 2 Coconut Peanut Butter Protein Bites (page 59)
Happy hour with colleagues and friends	Drinks, nachos, fries, food not ordered by you	Soda water with lemon An appetizer that includes vegetables, such as a hummus platter Shrimp cocktail Make the conscious decision to wait until you get home to eat
I like to unwind at night with a treat	Ice cream, cookies, chips	Nondairy plain yogurt with 1 tablespoon of walnuts and 1 teaspoon of honey Chocolate Chia Pudding Parfaits (page 52) Secret Ingredient Chocolate Mousse (page 56) Everything Seasoned Kale Chips (page 57)
I like to unwind at night with a drink	Red wine, white wine, beer, hard liquor	Sparkling water with a splash of cranberry juice Warming Bedtime Latte (page 63)
Treats at the office	Candy jar, homemade cookies	Pack your lunch so you're never starving Keep smart snacks available at your desk, like whole fruit, vegetables, and Coconut Peanut Butter Protein Bites (page 59)

Strategies for Socializing

Socializing might be the big challenge as you embark on this journey. The reality is, though, that for the rest of your life you'll be faced with social situations where you need to navigate food choices. It's my job to educate you on how to manage these situations successfully. Putting strategies in place *before* you face temptations will help you stick to your plan.

Take for instance a birthday celebration at the office where the default treat will be cake. Decide now to decline but also be ready with an explanation. Of course, you don't owe anyone an explanation and simply saying, "No, thanks—I don't want a slice of cake right now" *should* be enough. But we also know that's not always the case. "No, thanks—my body needs a little break from sugar at the moment" works great.

For restaurants, planning ahead by reviewing the menus before you walk through the doors is key. Once you're staring at a plate of nachos on the table next to you, it will be harder to choose the Cobb salad with the dressing on the side. But, if you already know what the temptations might be, then you can commit to a sensible choice that's in line with the detox diet. And once it's

in front of you, the salad will feel like a satisfying option, and you'll leave feeling proud of yourself, which matters just as much as the food you choose.

Building in the Time to Prep

Meal planning and prep work are two of the best things you can do for your future self. Carving out a small chunk of time each week (Sundays are popular) to plan your meals for the week and also make some things ahead of time will set you up for success as the week unfolds. Knowing in advance what you're making and what you're eating will give you peace of mind.

I've started you off by building out two weeks of meals and snacks. You can use that plan as a template. Feel free to swap out and move a meal around to make it work for you. At the start of each week, look over the recipes and see what you can make ahead of time.

Use your freezer; cook in bulk. If you're going through the effort of making the Everyday Pasta Sauce (page 135), double the recipe and freeze half for the next time you make a Bolognese sauce. Make your meal prep enjoyable, dedicate an afternoon, do it with family or recruit a friend, and stock your refrigerator so you're set for the week ahead.

The Meal Plan, Week 1

The following meal plans feature breakfast, lunch, dinner, and snack options. You'll see I have two snack options for each day, as you'll likely be reaching for one at some point between meals or after dinner. The snacks are always optional, and you can have one or both. The meals are balanced with protein, fat, and carbohydrates in an attempt to leave you feeling satisfied. Green vegetables are unlimited, so if you need more volume to your meals, add it there. And note that "side of fruit" means one whole fruit, such as an apple, orange, or pear, or 1 cup of berries (avoid bananas these 14 days, unless a recipe specifies).

And finally, if you find you're still very hungry after meals, try increasing your protein. To save you time and effort, some of the meals will use leftovers from prior meals; I have tried to indicate where that is the case, but you should feel free to improvise on that front.

> ▶ **Free Printables!**
>
> If you want to bring these to the grocery store or stick them on your fridge, these meal plans and shopping lists (plus the blank one on page 32) are available online at CallistoMediaBooks.com/14daydetox.

START A JOURNAL

Most people have the best success with clean eating when they track their intake. I'm not saying you need to spell out every single calorie, but writing down what you actually eat for breakfast, lunch, and dinner might help you make a smarter choice. For example, you were about to grab an apple but looking at your journal, you notice you already had two pieces of fruit earlier in the day, so instead you choose beef jerky or raw almonds.

You'll also want to keep track of days where you felt full and satisfied from recipes, of meals that left you a bit hungrier or wanting more, or of challenging circumstances you faced, etc. Short notes each day can also help keep you centered, reminding you how you got here, what your goals are, and what you're hoping to achieve.

week 1

	SUNDAY	MONDAY	TUESDAY
BREAKFAST	Easy Egg Frittata with Sun-Dried Tomatoes and Artichokes (page 80); any leftovers can be used Monday Roasted sweet potatoes Bacon (optional) Fruit	Blues and Greens Smoothie (page 39)	Protein-Packed Power Oatmeal (page 41)
LUNCH	Simple Homemade Hummus (page 53); any leftovers can be used Monday Raw vegetables for dipping	Leftover Easy Egg Frittata Side salad with Champagne Vinaigrette Apple	Tuna Salad in Romaine Lettuce Boats (page 68); any leftovers can be used Thursday Side of strawberries
SNACK	1 cup of yogurt with berries Apple with 1 tablespoon of almond butter Matcha Latte (page 62)	100-calorie pack almonds Leftover Simple Homemade Hummus Crunchy veggies of choice (cucumber, carrots, celery, etc.)	½ avocado with sea salt and lime Crunchy veggies of choice (cucumber, carrots, celery, etc.)
DINNER	Garlicky Green Turkey Meatballs (page 97) Easy Roasted Spaghetti Squash (page 138); any leftovers can be used Tuesday Everyday Pasta Sauce (page 135) Simple green salad with Champagne Vinaigrette (page 131); any leftovers can be used Monday	Sheet Pan Chicken Fajitas (page 99); any leftover chicken can be used Wednesday Cauliflower rice	Roasted Tomatoes with Shrimp (page 88) over leftover Easy Roasted Spaghetti Squash; any leftover shrimp can be used Wednesday Mediterranean Butter Lettuce Salad (page 70)

WEDNESDAY	THURSDAY	FRIDAY	SATURDAY
Jammy Peanut Butter Smoothie (page 38)	2 hard-boiled eggs 1 cup nondairy yogurt with ½ cup of berries	Protein-Packed Power Oatmeal (page 41)	Improvise brunch! Egg dish with veggies and avocado; add meat and/or potato if desired (no bread) Iced or hot unsweetened almond milk latte
You pick: leftover Chicken Fajita Bowl or salad with leftover shrimp	Leftover Tuna Salad in Romaine Lettuce Boats (page 68) Matcha Latte (page 62) over ice	Simple green salad with ½ avocado, 2 hard-boiled eggs, and Champagne Vinaigrette (page 131) Or leftovers of choice Piece of fruit	Snack/meal leftovers Clear out any leftovers from the week to start fresh on Sunday!
2 Coconut Peanut Butter Protein Bites (page 59) Apple with 1 tablespoon of nut butter	Jammy Peanut Butter Smoothie (page 38)	Chocolate Chia Pudding Parfaits (page 52); leftovers to be used Saturday	Piece of fruit Everything Seasoned Kale Chips (page 57) or Chocolate Chia Pudding Parfaits (page 52)
Green Soup (page 73) Warming Bedtime Latte (page 63)	Baked Lemon White Fish with Asparagus, Tomatoes, and Kalamata Olives (page 91)	Golden Roasted Chicken and White Beans (page 96) Sautéed spinach or kale	Flank Steak with Mushrooms and Baby Bok Choy (page 121); any leftovers to be used Monday Cauliflower rice, roasted broccoli, or green salad

shopping list

CANNED AND BOTTLED ITEMS

PANTRY ITEMS

- Artichoke hearts, water-packed, 2 (8-ounce) cans

- Cannellini beans, 1 (15-ounce) can

- Chickpeas, 1 (15-ounce) can

- Hearts of palm (1 can)

- Tomatoes, crushed, 1 (28-ounce) can

- Tuna, water-packed skipjack, 2 (5-ounce) cans

- Almond butter

- Almonds, 100-calorie packs (1 box)

- Avocado oil mayonnaise

- Capers

- Chia seeds

- Chicken stock, 1 (32-ounce) container

- Coconut, unsweetened shredded

- Flaxseed, ground

- Hemp hearts

- Kalamata olives

- Matcha powder

- Monk fruit sweetener

- Oats, rolled

- Peanut butter, natural

- Pistachios, salted roasted

- Protein powder, plant-based, vanilla

- Seasoning, taco

- Seasoning, everything bagel

- Sun-dried tomatoes, dry-pack (2 cups)

- Tahini

- Tamari

- Vegetable broth, 2 (32-ounce) containers

- Vinegar, champagne

PRODUCE

- Apples (5)
- Asparagus (1 bunch)
- Avocados (5)
- Baby carrots (1 package)
- Baby cucumbers (1 package)
- Bananas (1)
- Basil (1 bunch)
- Bell peppers, any color (3)
- Blueberries (1 pint)
- Bok choy, baby (8)
- Broccoli (2 heads)
- Butternut squash (1)
- Celery (1 head)
- Garlic (2 or 3 bulbs)
- Kale, chopped (12-ounce bag)
- Lemons (2)
- Lettuce, Bibb (2 heads)
- Lettuce, romaine (2 bags)
- Limes (2)
- Mushrooms, white, sliced (8 ounces)
- Onions, red (2)
- Onion, white (1)
- Parsley (1 bunch)
- Potatoes, mini, purple (1 pound)
- Raspberries (1 half-pint)
- Shallot (1)
- Spaghetti squash (1)
- Strawberries (1 quart)
- Sweet potatoes (2 medium)
- Tomatoes, cherry (4 pints)

DAIRY, EGGS, AND REFRIGERATED

- Almond milk, unsweetened (56 ounces)
- Nondairy milk, unsweetened (24 ounces)
- Eggs (1½ dozen)
- Liquid egg whites (16 ounces)
- Salsa, fresh (16 ounces)
- Yogurt, nondairy, unsweetened (24 ounces)

CONTINUED

shopping list continued

FROZEN

- Blueberries (12 ounces)
- Cauliflower, riced (two 10-ounce bags)
- Edamame, shelled (10 ounces)
- Raspberries (1 bag)
- Spinach (16 ounces)

MEAT, POULTRY, AND FISH

- Chicken breasts, boneless, skinless (1 pound)
- Chicken thighs, bone-in, skin-on (3 pounds)
- Flank steak (2 pounds)
- Haddock fillets (2 pounds)
- Shrimp, peeled and deveined, medium (1 pound)
- Turkey, ground (1 pound)

▶ **Check your pantry for these items:** balsamic vinegar, cinnamon, olive oil cooking spray, cumin, Dijon mustard, honey, maple syrup, oils (including extra-virgin olive, coconut, and avocado oils), onion salt, pepper, sea salt, turmeric, unsweetened cocoa powder, vanilla extract, and Worcestershire sauce

Advance Prep

With a busy schedule, it's easy to compromise and eat food that doesn't support your goals. To avoid compromising, I suggest you carve out around 2 hours on Sunday and prep the following:

- Easy Egg Frittata with Sun-Dried Tomatoes and Artichokes (page 80)
- Simple Homemade Hummus (page 53)
- Wash and chop celery, cucumber, carrots
- Garlicky Green Turkey Meatballs (page 97)
- Easy Roasted Spaghetti Squash (page 138)
- Everyday Pasta Sauce (page 135)
- Champagne Vinaigrette (page 131)
- Hard-boil 6 eggs to have on hand for snacks and meals

You'll also want to look ahead for the next day or two in the evening of the day prior. Can you prep enough breakfast, lunch, or snacks for the next two days? Looking ahead will allow you to be prepared as you head into the following day. It may feel like a bit of work initially, but the results will prove worth the effort.

week 2

	SUNDAY	MONDAY	TUESDAY
BREAKFAST	Green Eggs and Ham Breakfast Muffins (page 44); leftovers to be used Wednesday Fruit	Get Up and Go Smoothie (page 40)	Fruity Yogurt Parfait (page 45)
LUNCH	Kale Salad with Herby Chickpea "Croutons" (page 66); any leftover chickpeas to be used Monday; leftover kale salad to be used Wednesday	Romaine/mixed greens with leftover flank steak, berries, avocado, and Champagne Vinaigrette (page 131); leftover vinaigrette can be used Thursday	Chicken Salad with Walnuts, Grapes, and Celery (page 69)
SNACK	Secret Ingredient Chocolate Mousse (page 56); leftovers to be used Tuesday	Leftover Herby Roasted Chickpeas 1 cup of nondairy plain yogurt with ½ cup of berries	2 hard-boiled eggs Secret Ingredient Chocolate Mousse (page 56) 100-calorie pack almonds
DINNER	Sunday Lemon-Garlic Roast Chicken (page 101) Roasted sweet potato, cauliflower, and carrots Side salad	Buddha Bowls (page 85) with Crispy Tofu (page 140); leftover tofu can be used Wednesday	Grilled Turkey Burgers with Mango and Avocado (page 104); leftover turkey burger may be used Wednesday

WEDNESDAY	THURSDAY	FRIDAY	SATURDAY
2 Green Eggs and Ham Breakfast Muffins (page 44) ½ avocado or one piece of fruit	Smoothie of choice	Smoothie of choice	Almond Flour Waffles (page 48) 1 or 2 eggs prepared your choice
Leftover Kale Salad topped with baked tofu or turkey burger	Salad topped with salmon, mango, avocado, walnuts, and Champagne Vinaigrette (page 131)	Leftover pork with salad Side of fruit	Snack/meal leftovers Clear out any leftovers from the week to start fresh on Sunday!
Apple with 1 tablespoon of peanut butter	Fruity Yogurt Parfait (page 45) 100–calorie pack almonds	100–calorie pack mixed nuts/almonds	Piece of fruit Everything Seasoned Kale Chips (page 57) or Chocolate Chia Pudding Parfaits (page 52)
Foil Pack Salmon with Lemon Asparagus and Dairy-Free Tzatziki (page 90); leftover salmon can be used Thursday; leftover tzatziki can be used Saturday	Salsa Verde Shredded Pork and Kale (page 117); leftover pork to be used Friday	Hometown Crab Cakes (page 92) Roasted zucchini, onion, and summer squash	Slow-Roasted Lamb and Green Beans (page 127) Leftover Dairy-Free Tzatziki

shopping list

CANNED AND BOTTLED ITEMS

- Chickpeas, 1 (15-ounce can)
- Salsa verde, 1 (16-ounce bottle)
- Tomato sauce, 1 (8-ounce can)
- Tomatoes, crushed, 1 (28-ounce can)

PANTRY ITEMS

- Almond flour
- Herbes de Provence
- Old Bay seasoning
- Panko, gluten-free (1 bag)
- Quinoa (1 bag)
- Walnuts (1 bag)

PRODUCE

- Apples (3)
- Asparagus (2 bunches)
- Avocados (8)
- Bananas (1)
- Beans, green (1½ pounds)
- Bell pepper, green (1)
- Bell pepper, red (1)
- Berries of choice (1 pint)
- Broccoli (2 large stalks)
- Carrots, large (1 package)
- Celery (1 package)
- Cucumber (1)
- Dill (1 bunch)
- Garlic bulbs (2)
- Grapes (1 small bunch)
- Kale, chopped (four 10-ounce bags)
- Lemons (6)
- Lettuce, iceberg (1 head)
- Lettuce, romaine (2 heads)
- Lime (1)
- Mango (1)
- Mint (1 bunch)
- Onion, red (1)
- Onion, yellow (1)
- Parsley (1 bunch)
- Potatoes, small red (1 pound)
- Raspberries (1 half-pint)
- Sweet potatoes, medium (6)

DAIRY AND EGGS	FROZEN	MEAT, POULTRY, AND FISH

DAIRY AND EGGS

- Almond milk, unsweetened (24 ounces)
- Cold brew, unsweetened (2 cans or 1 bottle)
- Eggs (1½ dozen)
- Liquid egg whites (16 ounces)
- Tofu, extra-firm (12 ounces)
- Yogurt, nondairy, plain (36 ounces)

FROZEN

- Berries, of choice (1 bag)
- Cauliflower, riced (1 bag)
- Zucchini, chopped (10 ounces)

MEAT, POULTRY, AND FISH

- Chicken breasts, boneless, skinless (2)
- Chicken, whole (5 pounds)
- Crabmeat, jumbo lump, fresh (2 pounds)
- Ham, deli-sliced (½ pound)
- Lamb shoulder chops, boneless (3 pounds)
- Pork shoulder, boneless, or tenderloin (3 pounds)
- Salmon, 4 (6-ounce fillets)
- Turkey, ground (1 pound)

▶ **Things you should still have on hand from Week 1:** Almond butter, peanut butter, slivered almonds, chia seeds, hemp hearts, ground flaxseeds, tahini, champagne vinegar, tamari, everything bagel seasoning, protein powder, mayonnaise, monk fruit sweetener, and 100-calorie packs of almonds

▶ **Also check your pantry for:** Baking powder, cinnamon, unsweetened cocoa powder, olive oil cooking spray, ground ginger, maple syrup, oil (extra-virgin olive and avocado), pepper, sea salt, vanilla extract, and Worcestershire sauce

Advance Prep

Just as I mentioned previously, a little time to meal prep will be worth the effort. I suggest you carve out around 2 hours and prepare the following:

- Green Eggs and Ham Breakfast Muffins (page 44). You can freeze half for the future.

- Secret Ingredient Chocolate Mousse (page 56); Make sure you buy ripe avocados

- Cook 1 to 2 cups of dried quinoa according to the package directions

- Kale Salad with Herby Chickpea "Croutons" (page 66)

- Champagne Vinaigrette (page 131)

- Creamy Lemon-Tahini Dressing (page 132)

- Chopped and washed produce

- Optional: premake one of the smoothies

Beyond the 14-Day Plan

If you made it through the 14 days, I'm proud of you, but more important, you should be proud of yourself for committing the time and following through. I hope that you feel better physically and mentally than when you started, because you've been nourishing your body with healthy, whole foods. So now what?

I challenge you to keep following a meal plan that's close in structure to the past two weeks. I'm confident that you'll have started to notice so many positive changes that you'll be inspired to keep making better-for-you choices when it comes to food. And I'm hopeful that you recognize that making these choices isn't quite as difficult as you once thought it might be.

How to Reintroduce Foods

As you come out of the detox, remember to start slow, start small, plan ahead, and keep writing in your journal! Once the reins of the detox are off, it's easy to feel like you want to go hog wild, but don't. Reintroduction should be a methodical process.

For main food groups, start by adding back some dairy (if you plan to reintroduce it). Add plain yogurt into your meal or snack plan. Use cheese sparingly if you need it. If you feel okay, then you can move on to gluten. Make a note of how you feel after you eat one of the foods that you avoided for the last few weeks.

You're also likely itching to start indulging in some of the treats you missed the most and perhaps a glass of wine. You can—just keep portions in check and continue recording your intake to keep you honest and on track. This should probably look like a single

5-ounce glass of wine or 1 to 2 ounces of dark chocolate, ½ cup of ice cream or a mini candy bar. Be realistic and don't cheat yourself, but I encourage you to remember to keep healthy snacking options on hand for when you're feeling the urge to indulge.

You'll continue to notice trends on how certain foods make you feel and you'll probably start to make better-for-you choices just because they make you feel better, not because it's what the detox told you to choose.

Keep the Momentum Going

You can set yourself up for even more success by continuing to make a meal plan for every week. I've included a blank plan for you here to help you maintain the momentum that you've got going. Use this blank plan to make sure most of your meals follow the same guidelines as the meals in this book: a balance of protein, healthy fats, and complex carbohydrates. I'm sure many of the recipes from this book will even make it into your regular rotation.

But don't be afraid to include a meal that's a treat and a departure every now and again. Knowing that there's a pizza dinner to look forward to at the end of the week can help you stick to better choices on the other six nights. Remember, it's about progress, not perfection. When you plan for the vast majority of your meal choices to support your goals, you'll know that treating yourself won't derail all of your progress.

meal plan
worksheet

	SUNDAY	MONDAY	TUESDAY
BREAKFAST			
LUNCH			
SNACK			
DINNER			

The 14-Day Detox for Weight Loss

WEDNESDAY	THURSDAY	FRIDAY	SATURDAY

shopping list

CANNED AND BOTTLED ITEMS	PANTRY ITEMS	PRODUCE

DAIRY AND EGGS	FROZEN FOODS	MEAT & SEAFOOD

3

Breakfast

Jammy Peanut Butter Smoothie

Fast, Vegan

One sip of this smoothie and you'll be transported to the peanut butter and jelly sandwiches of your childhood. It is a win for our entire family and a weekday staple in our house. Feel free to make it the night before so you can grab and go on busy mornings. The consistency will be a bit thinner, but give it a good shake and it will still be great!

SERVES 1   *Prep time: 5 minutes*

1½ cups unsweetened almond milk

½ cup whole strawberries (3 or 4), fresh or frozen

1 cup baby spinach

1 tablespoon natural peanut butter

1 tablespoon ground flaxseed

1 scoop plant-based vanilla protein powder (with 20 to 25g protein per scoop)

4 or 5 ice cubes

In a blender, combine the almond milk, strawberries, spinach, peanut butter, ground flax, protein powder, and ice and blend on high until smooth.

Substitution tip: Swap out the strawberries for any other berry of your liking.

Cooking tip: If the smoothie is too thick, add up to ¼ cup of additional almond milk to reach your desired consistency.

Per Serving: Calories: 346; Fat: 16g; Saturated Fat: 1g; Cholesterol: 0mg; Carbohydrates: 22g; Fiber: 9.5g; Protein: 30g; Sodium: 714mg

Blues and Greens Smoothie

Fast, Vegan

Although the greens pack this smoothie with fiber, healthy fats, and protein to keep you going all morning long, their flavor takes a serious back seat to the full flavors of the banana, berries, and almond butter.

SERVES 1   *Prep time: 5 minutes*

1½ cups unsweetened almond milk

¼ cup fresh or frozen blueberries

¼ cup frozen banana slices

2 cups baby spinach or kale

1 tablespoon almond butter

1 tablespoon chia seeds

1 scoop plant-based vanilla protein powder (with 20 to 25g protein per scoop)

4 or 5 ice cubes

In a blender, combine the almond milk, blueberries, banana, spinach, almond butter, chia seeds, protein powder, and ice and blend on high until smooth.

Cooking tip: Any of the smoothies can be made the night before—they'll have a slightly thinner texter, but still taste great. Simply make as instructed the night before, cover and refrigerate, then shake before drinking.

Variation tip: Chocolate lovers can add 1 tablespoon of unsweetened cocoa powder to this delicious smoothie.

Per Serving: Calories: 411; Fat: 19g; Saturated Fat: 1.5g; Cholesterol: 0mg; Carbohydrates: 33g; Fiber: 15g; Protein: 33g; Sodium: 738mg

Get Up and Go Smoothie

Fast, Vegan

Here's your new frozen coffee drink, only without the expense, the line, or the unhealthy ingredients! Coffee and cocoa flavors pair nicely, and while frozen zucchini or cauliflower might sound weird, they will make the smoothie thick and creamy (plus add fiber!) without changing the flavor.

SERVES 1 *Prep time: 5 minutes*

½ cup unsweetened almond milk

½ cup brewed and cooled strong coffee or cold brew

1 tablespoon almond butter

1 small banana, frozen and cut into chunks

1 cup frozen chopped zucchini or riced cauliflower

1 tablespoon unsweetened cocoa powder

2 tablespoons hemp hearts or 1 scoop plant-based vanilla protein powder

1 teaspoon ground cinnamon

5 ice cubes (see Tip)

In a blender, combine the almond milk, coffee, almond butter, banana, zucchini, cocoa, hemp hearts, cinnamon, and ice and blend on high until smooth.

Cooking tip: Freeze leftover morning coffee in ice cube trays to use in your smoothie or to keep your homemade iced coffee from getting watered down.

Per Serving: Calories: 349; Fat: 20g; Saturated Fat: 2.5g; Cholesterol: 0mg; Carbohydrates: 5g; Fiber: 9.5g; Protein: 14g; Sodium: 135mg

Protein-Packed Power Oatmeal

Fast, Vegetarian

Oats are great for you, delivering a powerful boost of fiber and antioxidants. But sometimes a bowl of oatmeal isn't as filling as you'd like it to be. By whisking in some egg whites here, you'll get a fluffy, protein-packed, cozy bowl of oatmeal that will help you stay full long after eating. Try it topped with fruit.

SERVES 1   *Prep time: 2 minutes / Cook time: 7 minutes*

½ cup old-fashioned rolled oats

½ cup unsweetened almond milk

½ cup water

½ teaspoon vanilla or almond extract

½ teaspoon ground cinnamon

¼ cup liquid egg whites or 2 large egg whites

½ cup fresh or frozen raspberries

2 tablespoons slivered almonds

1 teaspoon almond butter

1. In a small saucepan, combine the oats, almond milk, water, vanilla, and cinnamon and cook over medium-low heat until the oats are tender and have mostly absorbed the liquid, about 5 minutes. Stir occasionally to prevent the oats from sticking.

2. Toward the end of the 5 minutes, whisk in the egg whites, whisking constantly for 1 to 2 minutes. This will prevent the eggs from scrambling but still allow them to cook through.

3. Pour into a bowl and top with the raspberries and almonds and drizzle with the almond butter.

Per Serving: Calories: 293; Fat: 11g; Saturated Fat: 1g; Cholesterol: 0mg; Carbohydrates: 38g; Fiber: 10g; Protein: 12g; Sodium: 152mg

Simple Broccoli-Avocado Omelet

Fast, Vegetarian

Omelets are so simple to make and come together quickly. I recommend broccoli and avocado here because I love how filling broccoli is, but any type of green vegetable would be great. Jarred salsa kicks up the flavor, as would any fresh herbs you have on hand.

SERVES 1 · *Prep time: 5 minutes / Cook time: 5 minutes*

½ cup liquid egg whites or 4 large egg whites

1 large egg

¼ teaspoon sea salt

¼ teaspoon freshly ground black pepper

2 teaspoons extra-virgin olive oil or olive oil cooking spray

1 cup frozen chopped broccoli, thawed

⅓ medium avocado, sliced

2 tablespoons salsa

1. In a small bowl, whisk together the egg whites, whole egg, salt, and pepper.

2. In a small nonstick skillet, heat the oil over medium-low heat so it coats the pan. Pour in the egg mixture and allow it to set for 3 to 4 minutes, running a soft spatula around the edges of the pan occasionally and tilting the pan so the liquid egg runs to the sides to set.

3. Once the omelet is almost set, spoon the broccoli and avocado on top of half of the omelet. Using a thin spatula, flip the uncovered half over the other side. (It's okay if this is not perfect!)

4. Slide the omelet out of the pan and top it with salsa.

Cooking tip: This is a perfect recipe to make with leftover broccoli or other green vegetables.

Per Serving: Calories: 320; Fat: 21g; Saturated Fat: 4g; Cholesterol: 186mg; Carbohydrates: 10g; Fiber: 6g; Protein: 17g; Sodium: 981mg

Butternut-Kale Breakfast Hash

Vegan, Nut-Free

Hash actually originated as a way to finish up leftovers, but this is not your average hash. The combination of caramelized squash, crispy kale, and soft, sweet apple blend nicely together for a luxurious weekend brunch. While the hash can be eaten alone, it is really delicious when topped with an egg or sautéed tofu.

SERVES 4   *Prep time: 10 minutes / Cook time: 30 minutes*

4 cups cubed peeled butternut squash or sweet potato

1 onion, diced

2 tablespoons extra-virgin olive oil

1 teaspoon sea salt

2 teaspoons smoked paprika

8 to 10 cups chopped kale (or a 16-ounce bag prechopped kale)

2 Granny Smith apples, peeled and diced

1. Preheat the oven to 400°F.

2. In a 10-inch cast-iron skillet or a baking dish, toss the squash and onion with the oil, salt, and paprika. Transfer to the oven and roast for 20 minutes.

3. Stir the squash mixture so it browns evenly, add the chopped kale and apple, toss, and return it to the oven roast until all ingredients are softened and caramelized, an additional 10 minutes.

Variation tip: This meal rounds out nicely with a poached or fried egg on top. Keep the yolk soft to soak up all the flavors.

Per Serving: Calories: 238; Fat: 8g; Saturated Fat: 1g; Cholesterol: 0mg; Carbohydrates: 40g; Fiber: 9.5g; Protein: 7g; Sodium: 632mg

Green Eggs and Ham Breakfast Muffins

Nut-Free

Don't let busy weekday mornings derail your clean-eating efforts. Make a batch of these muffins on a weekend, let them cool, wrap them up, and stash them in the freezer. You can grab three and reheat them quickly in the microwave. Paired with a piece of fruit, it's a complete meal. Even better, these are so tasty, they'll be popular with the entire family!

MAKES 12 MUFFINS *Prep time: 15 minutes / Cook time: 30 to 35 minutes*

Olive oil cooking spray

6 large eggs

1 cup liquid egg whites or 8 large egg whites

½ teaspoon sea salt

½ teaspoon freshly ground black pepper

½ onion, finely chopped

1 green bell pepper, finely diced

8 ounces deli ham, diced

1. Preheat the oven to 350°F. Line 12 cups of a muffin tin with liners and coat the liners with cooking spray, or generously spray each cup.

2. In a medium bowl, whisk the whole eggs, egg whites, salt, and black pepper.

3. In a separate medium bowl, combine the onion, bell pepper, and ham.

4. Divide the vegetable and ham mixture evenly among the 12 cups. They should be about two-thirds full. Pour the egg mixture over the veggies and meat until the cups are filled to the top.

5. Bake until the eggs are set and the tops are golden, 30 to 35 minutes.

Substitution tip: If you want to use liquid eggs instead of the whole eggs, use ¼ cup of liquid eggs for every whole egg. So for this recipe you'll need 1½ cups of liquid eggs (in addition to the liquid egg whites, which you still need).

Per Serving (3 muffins): Calories: 193; Fat: 9g; Saturated Fat: 2.5g; Cholesterol: 302mg; Carbohydrates: 4g; Fiber: 0.5g; Protein: 23g; Sodium: 1,178mg

Fruity Yogurt Parfait

Fast, Vegan

Today you'll find loads of nondairy yogurt options—almond, coconut, oat—which can be nice replacements, and that boast a texture very similar to dairy yogurt. Because nondairy yogurt is often not as high in protein as its dairy counterpart, hemp hearts and an optional scoop of protein powder are added for a boost. The protein powder also adds flavor.

SERVES 2   *Prep time: 10 minutes*

1½ cups plain
nondairy yogurt

1 tablespoon plant-based
vanilla protein powder
(optional)

1 tablespoon ground
flaxseed

1 tablespoon hemp hearts

1 teaspoon ground
cinnamon

½ teaspoon vanilla extract

1 apple, chopped

2 tablespoons slivered
almonds

2 teaspoons
almond butter

1. In a small bowl, combine the yogurt, protein powder (if using), ground flax, hemp hearts, cinnamon, and vanilla and stir to combine.

2. Divide the mixture between two bowls. Top each yogurt bowl with apple and almonds and drizzle with the almond butter.

Substitution tip: If you can't find plain nondairy yogurt, choose a flavored one. Just check and make sure the sugar content is no greater than 9 grams per serving.

Per Serving: Calories: 263; Fat: 15g; Saturated Fat: 1g; Cholesterol: 0mg; Carbohydrates: 29g; Fiber: 9g; Protein: 8.5g; Sodium: 44mg

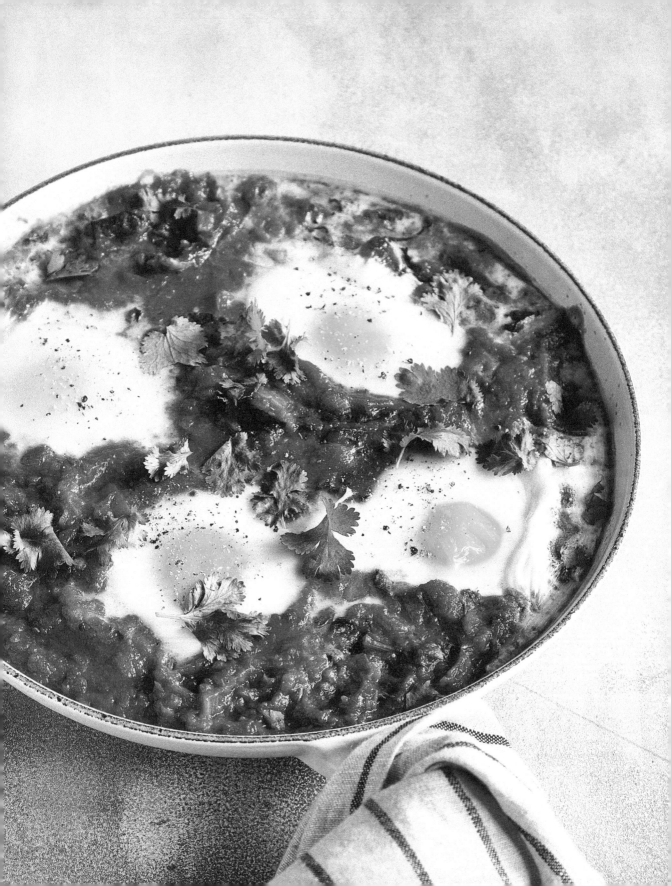

Easy Weekend Shakshuka

Vegetarian, Nut-Free

Shakshuka is a popular dish in the Middle East and North Africa. This hearty dish featuring baked eggs in a spiced tomato base is quite easy to make. It's excellent paired with fresh greens tossed with lemon, sliced avocado, and a side of roasted potato or sweet potato.

SERVES 4   *Prep time: 15 minutes / Cook time: 20 minutes*

2 tablespoons extra-virgin olive oil

1 cup diced onion

1 red bell pepper, diced

¼ teaspoon sea salt, plus more as needed

Freshly ground black pepper (optional)

2 garlic cloves, minced

2 tablespoons harissa or tomato paste

½ teaspoon smoked paprika

1 teaspoon ground cumin

1 (28-ounce) can crushed tomatoes

1 cup baby spinach, chopped

4 large eggs

¼ cup chopped fresh parsley or cilantro leaves, or both

1. Preheat the oven to 375°F.

2. In a 10- to 12-inch ovenproof skillet, heat the oil over medium heat. Add the onion, bell pepper, salt, and black pepper to taste (if using) and cook, stirring occasionally, until the vegetables begin to soften, 2 to 3 minutes.

3. Add the garlic, harissa, paprika, and cumin and stir again to coat everything. Add the tomatoes and let the mixture simmer for 10 minutes, stirring occasionally, to thicken the base and meld the flavors. Stir in the spinach.

4. Make 4 indentations in the sauce and crack an egg in the middle of each one.

5. Carefully place the skillet in the oven and bake until the eggs are set. You're looking for set whites, with yolks as runny as you desire, which takes 8 to 10 minutes. The eggs will continue to cook after you take the skillet out of the oven.

6. Top with fresh herbs and serve.

Ingredient tip: Harissa is a spicy pepper paste that is popular in the Middle East and North Africa. While not necessary, it adds a spicier profile than tomato paste to the dish.

Per Serving: Calories: 237; Fat: 12g; Saturated Fat: 2.5g; Cholesterol: 186mg; Carbohydrates: 21g; Fiber: 6.5g; Protein: 11g; Sodium: 667mg

Almond Flour Waffles

Fast, Vegetarian

Almond flour is a great grain-free flour option. It is lower in carbohydrates and higher in protein than the other more traditional flour options typically used in waffle recipes. Skip the traditional butter and syrup topping and instead top with seasonal fruit, nut butter, and/or nondairy yogurt to keep the sugar content low and your blood sugar stable.

MAKES ABOUT 6 WAFFLES *Prep time: 5 minutes / Cook time: 10 minutes*

3 large eggs

½ cup unsweetened nondairy milk

2 tablespoons avocado oil

1 teaspoon vanilla extract

2 cups blanched almond flour

½ teaspoon baking powder

Olive oil cooking spray

Fruit, nut butter, or nondairy yogurt, for topping

1. In a large bowl, whisk the eggs, milk, oil, and vanilla. Stir in the almond flour and baking powder.

2. Heat a waffle iron and coat with cooking spray. Cook the waffles according to the waffle iron directions. Place the cooked waffles on a baking sheet in a 300°F oven until you're ready to serve.

3. Top with your favorite toppings and enjoy!

Ingredient tip: The popularity of almond flour is on the rise, so you should have no trouble finding it in the baking section of any grocery store. Look for a "fine" or "super fine" blanched almond flour, which will yield the best results in baked goods.

Storage tip: Make a double batch of these and freeze the extra. Simply pop one into the toaster oven to reheat.

Per Serving (1 waffle without toppings): Calories: 319; Fat: 29g; Saturated Fat: 2.5g; Cholesterol: 93mg; Carbohydrates: 8g; Fiber: 3g; Protein: 11g; Sodium: 50mg

4

Snacks & Drinks

Chocolate Chia Pudding Parfaits

Vegan

This is an indulgent snack you can feel good about! You'll need to plan ahead for this rich and (seemingly) decadent chia pudding, as the chia seeds need time to gel, but it will be worth the wait. I like topping mine with nondairy yogurt and berries, but banana and a dollop of peanut butter are also amazing. Shredded, unsweetened coconut and cacao nibs take it to the next level.

SERVES 4   *Prep time: 10 minutes, plus overnight to set*

1½ cups unsweetened almond, cashew, or coconut milk

½ teaspoon vanilla extract

⅛ teaspoon sea salt

¼ cup unsweetened cocoa powder

½ cup chia seeds

1 to 2 tablespoons monk fruit sweetener

1 cup plain nondairy yogurt

1 cup mixed berries

1. In a small bowl, combine the milk, vanilla, salt, and cocoa powder. Whisk to combine, then add the chia seeds and whisk again to fully incorporate.

2. Add the monk fruit sweetener, starting with only 1 tablespoon and adding more a bit at a time until you reach your desired sweetness.

3. Cover and refrigerate for at least 4 hours or overnight.

4. Remove from the fridge and stir the mixture. It should have thickened because the chia seeds have expanded, resulting in a pudding-like consistency.

5. In 4 small jars or containers, layer the chia mixture with the yogurt and berries.

6. The parfaits will keep in the refrigerator for about 5 days.

Substitution tip: Don't have monk fruit sweetener? Use 2 or 3 drops of liquid stevia instead.

Per Serving: Calories: 206; Fat: 13g; Saturated Fat: 3g; Cholesterol: 0mg; Carbohydrates: 27g; Fiber: 15g; Protein: 6g; Sodium: 229mg

Simple Homemade Hummus

Fast, Vegan, Nut-Free

While store-bought hummus is convenient, making your own at home is worth doing: It's easy, the finished product tastes light and fresh, and there are no hidden ingredients. It's such a great snack to have on hand because you can pair it with crunchy vegetables to carry you until dinner or use it to add a little extra protein to a meal.

MAKES ABOUT 2 CUPS   *Prep time: 10 minutes*

1 (15-ounce) can chickpeas, drained and rinsed

¼ cup water

¼ cup tahini

3 tablespoons extra-virgin olive oil

1 garlic clove, minced

1 teaspoon sea salt

½ teaspoon ground cumin

2 tablespoons freshly squeezed lemon juice

1. In a food processor, pulse the chickpeas and water until the chickpeas start to break up and form a paste.

2. Add the tahini, oil, garlic, salt, cumin, and lemon juice and puree until smooth. Pause halfway through mixing to scrape down the sides and incorporate everything.

3. Serve immediately or cover and refrigerate for up to 5 days.

Cooking tip: If the hummus seems too thick, add another 1 to 2 tablespoons of water. If it seems a little thin, don't worry; it will thicken as it sits in the refrigerator.

Variation tip: This basic recipe can take on any flavor variation you wish. Delectable additions include smoked paprika, sun-dried tomatoes, or Kalamata olives.

Per Serving (¼ cup): Calories: 149; Fat: 10g; Saturated Fat: 1.5g; Cholesterol: 0mg; Carbohydrates: 12g; Fiber: 3g; Protein: 5g; Sodium: 380mg

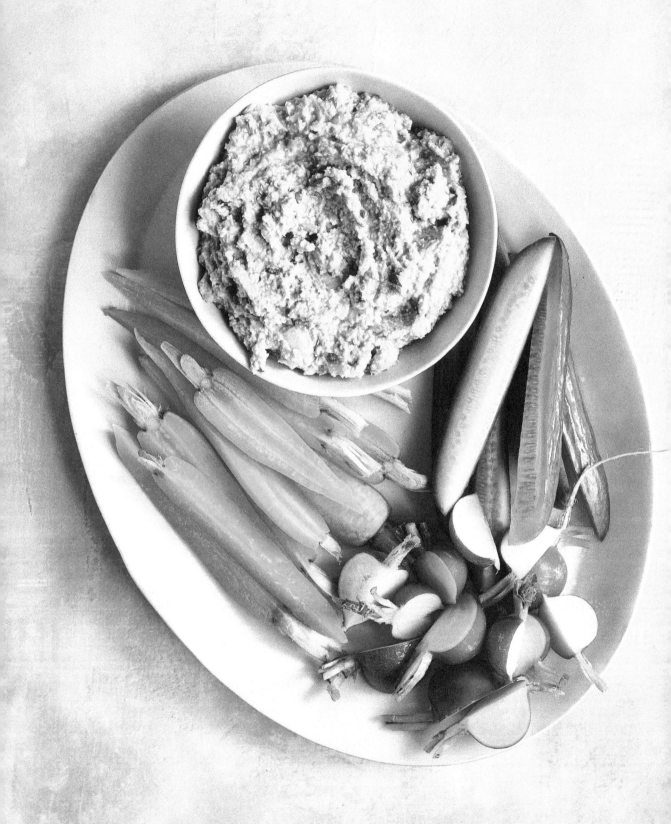

Edamame Guacamole

Fast, Vegan, Nut-Free

I love this spin on a classic favorite. Edamame adds a nice texture to the dip while also delivering a boost of protein, which you don't get from traditional guac. Use this dip as a snack paired with crunchy carrots, celery, and cucumber; as a topping on a salad; or as a sauce for a main dish like fish or chicken.

MAKES 1 CUP   *Prep time: 10 minutes / Cook time: 10 minutes*

1 cup frozen shelled edamame, thawed

2 tablespoons water, plus more as needed

1 avocado, halved and pitted

2 tablespoons freshly squeezed lime juice

¼ cup diced onion

½ cup chopped fresh cilantro

Sea salt

Freshly ground black pepper

1. Cook the edamame according to the package directions. Let cool.

2. In a food processor, combine the edamame and water and pulse until the edamame starts to break up.

3. Scoop the avocado into the processor, add the lime juice, and pulse again to incorporate. If the mixture seems very thick and a little dry, add more water, a tablespoon at a time, until you reach your desired consistency.

4. Transfer the mixture to a bowl and stir in the onion and cilantro. Season with salt and pepper to taste.

5. Serve immediately or cover and refrigerate up to 5 days.

Ingredient tip: Edamame are a great source of protein, and are also high in fiber and antioxidants. They make a great snack or addition to salads, soups, and more.

Per Serving (¼ cup): Calories: 113; Fat: 7g; Saturated Fat: 0.5g; Cholesterol: 0mg; Carbohydrates: 9g; Fiber: 4.5g; Protein: 5g; Sodium: 19mg

Secret Ingredient Chocolate Mousse

Vegan, Nut-Free

If you've never had chocolate mousse made with avocado, you're in for a really pleasant surprise. It doesn't taste like guacamole; the avocado just lends creaminess and "good" monounsaturated fat. Avocados can help stabilize your blood sugar (preventing spikes and crashes in energy), reduce cravings, and keep you full and satisfied. This sweet treat is a fun way to reap the benefits of avocado while still feeling like you're indulging.

SERVES 4 *Prep time: 5 minutes, plus 1 to 3 hours to chill*

2 avocados, halved and pitted

¼ cup unsweetened cocoa powder

1 tablespoon ground flaxseed

1 teaspoon vanilla extract

2 tablespoons pure maple syrup

2 tablespoons water, plus more as needed

Pinch sea salt

Monk fruit sweetener or liquid stevia for sweetening

Optional toppings: berries, cocoa nibs, coconut flakes, plain nondairy yogurt, or fresh mint

1. Scoop the avocados into a food processor and pulse two to three times until the avocados start to become pureed.

2. Add the cocoa powder, ground flax, vanilla, maple syrup, water, and salt and blend until smooth. If the mousse is too thick, add more water, 1 tablespoon at a time, until you reach your desired consistency.

3. Once blended, add the monk fruit to your desired sweetness level (less is more here).

4. Let chill for 1 to 3 hours in the refrigerator. The pudding will get thicker and richer in flavor as it sits.

5. Once chilled, divide into 4 servings. If desired, add your choice of toppings.

Per Serving (without toppings): Calories: 157; Fat: 11g; Saturated Fat: 1.5g; Cholesterol: 0mg; Carbohydrates: 16g; Fiber: 7g; Protein: 3g; Sodium: 7mg

Everything Seasoned Kale Chips

Fast, Vegan, Nut-Free

Known for being a great source of fiber, vitamin C, and calcium, kale is hearty and versatile. In this book, you'll find it in salads, soups, breakfast dishes, and here as "chips." Baking the kale makes it crisp and crunchy, and when you're craving a salty snack, these will do the trick.

SERVES 2   *Prep time: 5 minutes / Cook time: 20 minutes*

1 (12-ounce) bag chopped kale

2 tablespoons extra-virgin olive oil

1 tablespoon everything bagel seasoning

1. Preheat the oven to 300°F.
2. Spread the kale on a sheet pan. Drizzle on the oil and sprinkle with the everything bagel seasoning and toss to coat.
3. Bake until dried and crispy, checking after 10 minutes. If not crispy yet, return to the oven for another 5 to 10 minutes.
4. Eat immediately or store in a container at room temperature for 1 day. Note that chips may lose crispness as they sit.

Cooking tip: These can go from not-crispy-enough to burned-to-a-crisp really quickly, so keep a close eye on them!

Per Serving: Calories: 233; Fat: 15g; Saturated Fat: 2g; Cholesterol: 0mg; Carbohydrates: 17g; Fiber: 6g; Protein: 7g; Sodium: 455mg

Herby Roasted Chickpeas

Vegan, Nut-Free

Chickpeas are high in both protein and fiber, and also full of great vitamins and minerals, making them a really smart choice. When roasted like this, they become crispy and perfect for a midafternoon snack. They're also great on top of a lunchtime salad or as part of a plant-based dinner. Here, I'm using herbes de Provence, but any of your favorite spice combinations will work.

MAKES ABOUT 1¾ CUPS *Prep time: 10 minutes / Cook time: 30 to 40 minutes*

1 (15-ounce) can chickpeas, rinsed, drained, and patted dry

2 tablespoons extra-virgin olive oil

1 tablespoon herbes de Provence

½ teaspoon sea salt

1. Preheat the oven to 400°F.

2. In a medium bowl, toss together the chickpeas, oil, herbs, and salt. Spread them on a baking sheet in a single layer.

3. Bake until crisp, 30 to 40 minutes, shaking the pan midway through cooking.

Variation tip: Take the flavor up a notch by using 1 teaspoon of smoked paprika and ⅛ teaspoon of cayenne pepper in place of the herbes de Provence.

Per Serving (¼ cup): Calories: 87; Fat: 5g; Saturated Fat: 0.5g; Cholesterol: 0mg; Carbohydrates: 8g; Fiber: 2.5g; Protein: 3g; Sodium: 333mg

Coconut Peanut Butter Protein Bites

Vegan

This is a snack you're going to be happy to have on hand before or after a good workout. With the combination of oats, nut butter, and protein powder, these bites are ideal for an energy boost or regeneration. My only caveat: Indulge in no more than one or two at a time.

MAKES 8 BITES   *Prep time: 10 minutes, plus at least 20 minutes to chill*

2 tablespoons plant-based protein powder

⅔ cup old-fashioned rolled oats

¼ cup unsweetened shredded coconut

½ cup natural peanut butter

1 tablespoon water, plus more as needed

1 tablespoon cacao nibs (optional)

Pinch sea salt

1. In a food processor, combine the protein powder, oats, coconut, peanut butter, and water and blend until dough comes together. If the dough seems dry, add more water, 1 tablespoon at a time, until a dough forms. Once the dough reaches your desired consistency add the cacao nibs (if using) and salt and pulse a few more times to incorporate throughout.

2. Using a small ice-cream scoop (or spoon), portion the dough into 8 balls and refrigerate for at least 20 minutes or until ready to serve.

Ingredient tip: Cacao nibs are bits of pieces from cacao beans. While slightly bitter, they deliver tons of nutrients, including antioxidants and fiber. I also love how they add a really nice texture, the way chocolate chips would, but without any added sugar.

Variation tip: These bites are super versatile. Swap peanut butter for almond butter, add cocoa powder for a chocolate version, or slip in some pumpkin pie spice or cinnamon for some autumnal flair. The options are limitless!

Per Serving (2 bites): Calories: 310; Fat: 21g; Saturated Fat: 5.5g; Cholesterol: 0mg; Carbohydrates: 17g; Fiber: 4g; Protein: 12g; Sodium: 189mg

Crunchy Veggie Summer Rolls

Fast, Vegan

Fresh crunchy vegetables, buttery avocado, and bright herbs come together to make a light, fresh snack that can feel more satisfying than just a salad. Make sure your ingredients are thinly sliced for filling (a mandoline works great if you have one), and don't fret if your "wrapping" on these is not perfect. They'll still be delicious.

4 SERVINGS   *Prep time: 20 minutes*

4 (6-inch) rice paper rounds

4 romaine or green leaf lettuce leaves, midribs removed

1 avocado, thinly sliced

4 radishes, thinly sliced

½ cup shredded carrots

½ large red bell pepper, thinly sliced

8 to 10 fresh basil or mint leaves (optional)

For dipping (optional): tamari or Peanut Sauce (page 136)

1. Have all your prepped vegetables close at hand. Fill a shallow bowl or pie plate with warm water.

2. Gently dip a rice paper in the water and lay on a work surface, like a wooden cutting board. You'll notice the rice paper will go from stiff and paper-like to very pliable. They can get sticky, so don't leave them in the water too long. You can always dip your finger in the water and run it over the rice paper once it's lying flat on the board. (Expect a few mess ups!)

3. Cut the lettuce to the size of the rice wrapper and place on the near edge. Place a small amount of each of the vegetables (avocado, radishes, carrots, bell pepper) and herbs (if using) on top of the lettuce.

4. Starting from the side the lettuce is on, gently start rolling the wrapper. When you get to the middle, fold in the sides, burrito-style, and continue to wrap until it's fully closed. Place the finished rolls on a plate and set aside.

5. Repeat with the remaining rounds of rice paper and the rest of the vegetables.

6. Cut the rolls in half or eat them whole. If desired, serve with tamari or peanut sauce for dipping.

Ingredient tip: The basil or mint are optional ingredients here but really enhance the flavor profile and are well worth grabbing when you're at the market.

Variation tip: Make these rolls heartier by adding sliced cooked shrimp or tofu inside each one.

Per Serving: Calories: 115; Fat: 5.5g; Saturated Fat: 1g; Cholesterol: 0mg; Carbohydrates: 18g; Fiber: 4g; Protein: 2g; Sodium: 59mg

Matcha Latte

Fast, Vegan, Nut-Free

Matcha is a traditional Japanese green tea made from very finely ground tea leaves. The result is a flavor that can seem a bit bitter or "grassy," but is delicious in combination with other ingredients. It's gaining popularity thanks to its health benefits, so you've likely seen it at your local coffee shop. However, the coffee shop version is often sky-high in added sugar. This version combines nondairy milk, matcha tea powder, and protein powder to give you a flavorful drink that's free of any ingredients that might derail your clean-eating efforts.

1 SERVING   *Prep time: 5 minutes / Cook time: 3 minutes*

1½ cups unsweetened nondairy milk, warmed

1 teaspoon matcha powder

2 tablespoons plant-based vanilla protein powder or 2 drops liquid stevia

In a blender, combine the warmed milk, matcha powder, and protein powder and blend until frothy, 10 to 20 seconds. Pour into a mug and enjoy.

Ingredient tip: You can find matcha at all grocery stores today with the rest of the tea. The benefit of matcha over a bag of steeped green tea? It gives the body a gentler boost of caffeine in addition to a concentrated boost of antioxidants (far more than a steeped green tea bag) with health-protective benefits.

Per Serving: Calories: 99; Fat: 4.5g; Saturated Fat: 0g; Cholesterol: 0mg; Carbohydrates: 5g; Fiber: 3g; Protein: 9g; Sodium: 387mg

Warming Bedtime Latte

Fast, Vegetarian

This latte combines warming turmeric and cinnamon with vanilla, honey, and coconut, creating a cozy drink perfect for a nightcap. Turmeric is a vibrant orange spice you often see in curries, but its uses extend much further. Thanks to its main compound, curcumin, it's been used as medicine for thousands of years, and it has noted anti-inflammatory properties.

1 SERVING *Prep time: 2 minutes / Cook time: 3 minutes*

1½ cups unsweetened nondairy milk, such as almond milk

1 tablespoon honey

1 teaspoon coconut oil

1 teaspoon ground turmeric

1 teaspoon ground cinnamon

½ teaspoon vanilla extract

Pinch freshly ground black pepper

1. In a small saucepan, warm the milk over low heat. Whisk in the honey, coconut oil, turmeric, cinnamon, vanilla, and pepper.

2. In a blender, blend the warmed mixture until frothy. Pour into a mug and enjoy. (This step is optional, but it gives it a nice texture.)

Ingredient tip: Curcumin is absorbed best with the presence of black pepper, so make sure to keep that pinch in the recipe.

Per Serving: Calories: 155; Fat: 8g; Saturated Fat: 3.5g; Cholesterol: 0mg; Carbohydrates: 19g; Fiber: 1.5g; Protein: 2g; Sodium: 256mg

Salads & Soups

5

Kale Salad with Herby Chickpea "Croutons"

Fast, Vegan

Kale can be intense to eat raw, but when given a good massage, the leaves get tender and soft and it becomes a really delicious salad green. Also, because kale is such a sturdy green, this salad will keep for a few days for leftovers, but don't add the fresh fruit and crispy chickpeas until just before serving.

SERVES 4   *Prep time: 15 minutes*

1 (16-ounce) bag chopped kale (or 2 large bunches kale, ribs removed and leaves chopped)

½ teaspoon sea salt

½ teaspoon freshly ground black pepper

2 tablespoons freshly squeezed lemon juice

1 tablespoon extra-virgin olive oil

2 cups cooked quinoa, cooled (optional)

2 tablespoons Creamy Lemon-Tahini Dressing (page 132), divided

1 cup Herby Roasted Chickpeas (page 58)

½ cup fresh berries of your choice

1. Place the kale in a large bowl and sprinkle with the salt, pepper, lemon juice, and oil. Use your hands to gently "massage" the kale. Do this for a few minutes until you notice the leaves starting to soften. The oil and salt will help this process.

2. Once the leaves have softened, add the quinoa (if using) and 1 tablespoon of tahini dressing and toss.

3. Divide into four bowls and top with the chickpeas, berries, and a drizzle more of dressing, if desired.

4. Store leftover kale salad in an airtight container in the refrigerator for up to 4 days.

Ingredient tip: You can buy traditional curly kale, but the flat-leaf lacinato or Tuscan kale (sometimes called dinosaur kale) is a delicious option for this salad.

Per Serving: Calories: 207; Fat: 12g; Saturated Fat: 1.5g; Cholesterol: 0mg; Carbohydrates: 21g; Fiber: 8g; Protein: 8g; Sodium: 731mg

Roasted Vegetable Salad with Pesto Drizzle

Vegan

This is a warming salad for chilly days. It could be a main course for lunch or dinner; just add a poached egg for some extra protein, if needed. The wide array of colors, flavors, and textures make the prep and planning for this pretty salad worth it. If you don't have time to make pesto, look for a dairy-free store-bought version.

SERVES 2   *Prep time: 15 minutes / Cook time: 30 minutes*

2 (1-pound) delicata squash, sliced

½ pound Brussels sprouts (10 to 12), quartered

½ small head cauliflower, chopped

2 tablespoons extra-virgin olive oil, divided

1 apple, chopped

1 cup chopped cucumber

1 avocado, cubed

4 cups mixed greens, such as arugula, chopped kale, or baby spinach

1 teaspoon lemon juice or apple cider vinegar

Sea salt

Freshly ground black pepper

2 tablespoons Spinach-Walnut Pesto (page 137)

1. Preheat the oven to 400°F.

2. In a medium bowl, toss together the squash, Brussels sprouts, cauliflower, and 1 tablespoon of olive oil. Spread in a single layer on one or two sheet pans, depending on the size of your pans.

3. Roast until the vegetables are tender and slightly browned, 25 to 30 minutes, stirring once or twice.

4. Meanwhile, combine the apple, cucumber, and avocado in a bowl and refrigerate to keep cold. In a large, shallow bowl, toss the greens with the remaining 1 tablespoon olive oil, the lemon juice, and salt and pepper to taste.

5. Place the warm vegetables on top of the salad greens, followed by the crisp and cold cucumber, apple, and avocado.

6. Drizzle the salad with the pesto and serve.

Substitution tip: If you can't find delicata squash, which is usually seasonal in fall, swap out for butternut squash cubes or even sweet potato.

Per Serving: Calories: 534; Fat: 28g; Saturated Fat: 4g; Cholesterol: 0mg; Carbohydrates: 73g; Fiber: 20g; Protein: 12g; Sodium: 287mg

Tuna Salad in Romaine Lettuce Boats

Fast, Nut-Free

Packed with pure protein and healthy fats, this tuna will keep you full for hours. I love to wrap my tuna salad in crunchy romaine lettuce, but it's also very easy to throw on top of a salad or even pair with a side of roasted broccoli and potato wedges for a day when you want something a little warmer. I recommend skipjack tuna, which is the lowest in mercury, but any tuna packed in water is fine.

SERVES 2 *Prep time: 10 minutes*

2 (5-ounce cans) water-packed skipjack tuna, drained

1 tablespoon extra-virgin olive oil

1 tablespoon avocado oil mayonnaise

1 tablespoon freshly squeezed lemon juice (optional)

Optional add-ins:
1 teaspoon drained capers, 2 tablespoons finely chopped red onion, 2 tablespoons chopped fresh parsley, and/or 1 celery stalk, chopped

6 to 8 large romaine lettuce leaves

1. In a small bowl, combine the tuna, oil, and mayonnaise. Using a fork, flake the tuna to separate and combine with the ingredients.

2. Add the lemon juice (if using) and any or all of the optional add-ins and stir to combine.

3. If serving right away, spoon the salad onto romaine lettuce leaves. Or refrigerate covered for up to 3 days.

Ingredient tip: In addition to being mindful of mercury content when choosing your tuna, look for brands selling BPA-free cans with pole- and line-caught fish, a more sustainable process in which fish are caught one at a time.

Per Serving: Calories: 222; Fat: 13g; Saturated Fat: 1.5g; Cholesterol: 61mg; Carbohydrates: 2g; Fiber: 1.5g; Protein: 25g; Sodium: 485mg

Chicken Salad with Walnuts, Grapes, and Celery

Fast

Thanks to sweet grapes, crunchy walnuts, and celery, you get to indulge in a variety of textures and flavors with this chicken salad. It's so easy to make this using a store-bought rotisserie chicken or chicken from your Sunday leftovers. That said, if you don't have cooked chicken on hand, you can always poach or bake two chicken breasts for this recipe.

SERVES 4 *Prep time: 15 minutes*

¼ cup avocado oil mayonnaise

¼ cup plain nondairy yogurt

¼ cup chopped fresh parsley (optional)

½ teaspoon sea salt, or more as needed

½ teaspoon freshly ground black pepper, or more as needed

2 cups diced or shredded cooked chicken

½ cup chopped celery

¼ cup finely chopped red onion

½ cup seedless grapes, sliced

¼ cup chopped toasted walnuts

Mixed greens or romaine lettuce, for serving

In a large bowl, combine the mayonnaise, yogurt, parsley (if using), salt, and pepper. Stir in the chicken, celery, onion, grapes and walnuts, and add more salt and pepper if needed. Serve over a bed of greens or in romaine leaves.

Per Serving: Calories: 268; Fat: 18g; Saturated Fat: 2.5g; Cholesterol: 82mg; Carbohydrates: 6g; Fiber: 1g; Protein: 22g; Sodium: 727mg

Mediterranean Butter Lettuce Salad

Fast, Vegan

This salad is a great accompaniment to Italian-inspired dishes, like the Sneaky Veggie Bolognese (page 119) served over Easy Roasted Spaghetti Squash (page 138) or with Garlicky Green Turkey Meatballs (page 97).

SERVES 4   *Prep time: 10 minutes*

2 heads Bibb lettuce, chopped

1 (8-ounce) can artichoke hearts, chopped

2 cups sliced seeded cucumber

1 cup sliced hearts of palm

1 cup cherry tomatoes, halved

½ cup pitted Kalamata olives, chopped

1 cup sun-dried tomatoes, chopped

½ cup Champagne Vinaigrette (page 131)

½ cup salted roasted pistachios

In a large salad bowl, toss together the lettuce, artichoke hearts, cucumber, hearts of palm, cherry tomatoes, olives, sun-dried tomatoes, and vinaigrette. Sprinkle on the pistachios and serve.

Ingredient tip: Bibb or butter lettuce is a nice soft lettuce that pairs well with these ingredients. That said, don't fret if you can't find it. Any leafy green lettuce will work great.

Per Serving: Calories: 334; Fat: 24g; Saturated Fat: 2.5g; Cholesterol: 0mg; Carbohydrates: 25g; Fiber: 6.5g; Protein: 8g; Sodium: 1,180mg

Black Bean and Mango Salad

Fast, Vegan, Nut-Free

The combination of mango, black beans, corn, and avocado in this salad is delicious. It works perfectly in butter lettuce "cups," but also is a great side salad to serve with Salsa Verde Shredded Pork and Kale (page 117). You can bulk this up with lettuce or cooked quinoa if you like. For a pretty (and portable) presentation, layer the ingredients in a quart-size jar, starting with the heavier ingredients (like the beans) and working your way up. Decant it onto a plate or bowl and toss with the dressing before serving.

SERVES 2   *Prep time: 10 minutes*

2 tablespoons freshly squeezed lime juice

2 tablespoons extra-virgin olive oil

1 teaspoon ground cumin

½ teaspoon sea salt

½ teaspoon freshly ground black pepper

1 avocado, diced

1 cup fresh or frozen corn kernels, thawed

1 red bell pepper, diced

1 mango, diced

1 (15-ounce) can black beans, drained and rinsed

¼ cup chopped fresh cilantro

1. In a large bowl, whisk together the lime juice, oil, cumin, salt, and black pepper.

2. Add the avocado, corn, bell pepper, mango, beans, and cilantro and toss to combine.

Storage tip: This salad can be made ahead of time and stored in the refrigerator for up to 3 days. Don't add the avocado until just before serving.

Per Serving: Calories: 306; Fat: 13g; Saturated Fat: 2g; Cholesterol: 0mg; Carbohydrates: 43g; Fiber: 12g; Protein: 9g; Sodium: 459mg

Nana's Lentil Soup

Vegan, Nut-Free

Passed down from my great-grandmother Nana, generations of my family have made this soup. We all make a slightly different version, but the ingredients and simplicity of it are essentially the same. Lentils serve as the base; they are low in calories, high in protein, and a great plant-based source of iron and folate.

SERVES 6   *Prep time: 15 minutes / Cook time: 1 to 2 hours*

2 tablespoons extra-virgin olive oil

1 cup chopped carrots

1 cup chopped celery (with the leafy tops if you have them)

½ cup chopped yellow onion

2 garlic cloves, minced

1 teaspoon sea salt, plus more as needed

3 tablespoons tomato paste

1½ cups brown lentils, rinsed and picked over

4 cups vegetable broth

2 cups water, plus more as needed

4 to 6 cups baby spinach

Freshly ground black pepper

2 tablespoons freshly squeezed lemon juice or apple cider vinegar (optional)

1. In large stockpot, heat the oil over medium-high heat. Add the carrots, celery (including the tops), onion, garlic, and salt and sauté until the vegetables soften, 5 to 10 minutes.

2. Add the tomato paste and lentils and stir to incorporate.

3. Add the vegetable broth and water and bring to a boil over high heat. Boil for 5 minutes, then reduce the heat to medium-low and simmer until the lentils are tender and the soup has thickened, 40 to 50 minutes. (The longer and slower you simmer the soup, the more the flavors will blend and develop.)

4. Add the spinach right before serving so it wilts. Season with pepper to taste and a squeeze of lemon juice (if using). Taste and season with more salt if needed.

5. Serve or store covered in the refrigerator for 5 days or freeze for 3 months.

Cooking tip: Make this in your slow cooker. Add all ingredients and set on low to cook for 8 hours. Stir and add the spinach plus additional broth or water to thin the soup before serving, if you prefer.

Per Serving: Calories: 262; Fat: 5g; Saturated Fat: 1g; Cholesterol: 0mg; Carbohydrates: 42g; Fiber: 9g; Protein: 14g; Sodium: 842mg

Green Soup

Vegan, Nut-Free

I absolutely love this soup, both for its taste and for its versatility. Feel free to supplement or substitute with any ingredients you have on hand, such as fresh zucchini, kale, peas, or cauliflower. I usually have bags of frozen spinach, broccoli, and edamame in my freezer, which makes this soup come together in minutes but taste like it's been simmering for hours.

SERVES 4   *Prep time: 15 minutes / Cook time: 20 to 30 minutes*

2 tablespoons extra-virgin olive oil

3 garlic cloves

4 cups fresh or frozen chopped broccoli, thawed

½ teaspoon sea salt, or more as needed

½ teaspoon freshly ground black pepper, or more as needed

2 cups frozen shelled edamame

6 cups low-sodium vegetable broth or bone broth of choice

1 tablespoon freshly squeezed lemon juice

4 cups baby spinach or 1 to 2 cups frozen chopped spinach

2 avocados, diced

Handful chopped fresh herbs, such as basil, parsley, or cilantro (optional)

1. In a medium pot, heat the oil over medium heat. Add the garlic, broccoli, salt, and pepper and sauté until the broccoli becomes a bit tender, about 5 minutes.

2. Add the edamame and broth and bring to a boil over high heat, then reduce the heat to low and simmer for 10 to 15 minutes.

3. Add the lemon juice and spinach. If using frozen spinach, simmer for 5 to 10 minutes before serving. If using fresh spinach, serve immediately after adding.

4. Ladle the soup into bowls and top each bowl with avocado and fresh herbs (if using).

Ingredient tip: Feeling a cold coming on? Garlic has both antiviral and antimicrobial properties, and lemons are high in vitamin C, making this a great soup to whip up when you're feeling like you're coming down with something.

Per Serving: Calories: 357; Fat: 21g; Saturated Fat: 2.5g; Cholesterol: 0mg; Carbohydrates: 28g; Fiber: 14g; Protein: 13g; Sodium: 599mg

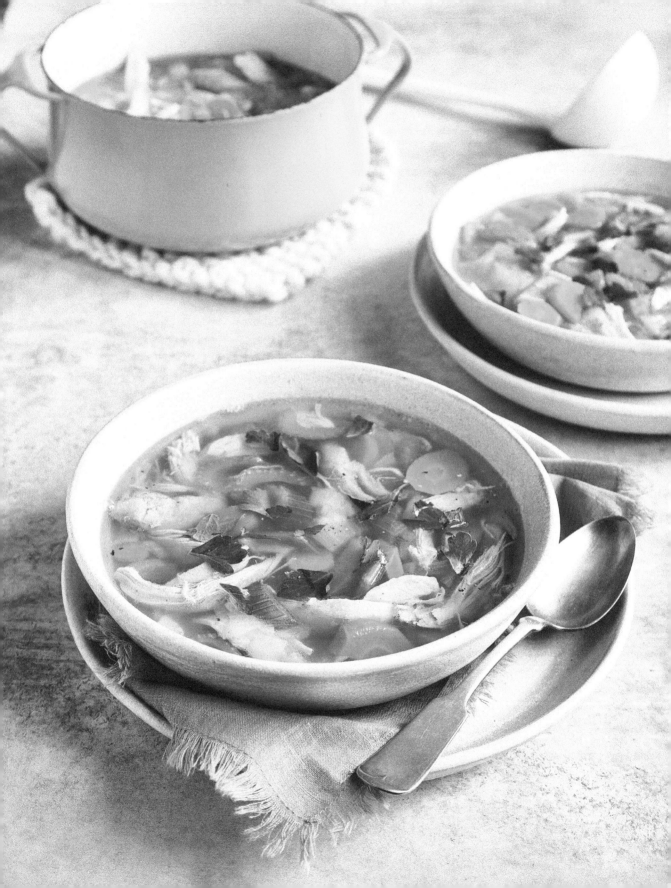

Quickest Chicken Soup

Fast, Nut-Free

This soup is made with bone broth, which is stock that comes from simmering bones and connective tissues. It is well worth the slightly higher price than traditional stock because not only is it richer in flavor, but it also delivers vitamins and minerals, amino acids (protein), and essential fatty acids.

SERVES 4 TO 6   *Prep time: 10 minutes / Cook time: 20 minutes*

2 tablespoons extra-virgin olive oil

1 medium onion, chopped

3 medium carrots, chopped

2 celery stalks, chopped

1 teaspoon sea salt, plus more as needed

3 garlic cloves, minced

1 rotisserie chicken, meat removed and shredded or chopped, skin and bones discarded

6 cups chicken bone broth

2 cups water

1 bay leaf

Juice of 1 lemon

Freshly ground black pepper

1. In a large pot, heat the oil over medium heat. Add the onion, carrots, celery, and salt and sauté until the onions become translucent and the vegetables start to soften, 4 to 5 minutes. Add the garlic and chicken and cook until the garlic is fragrant, about 1 minute.

2. Add the bone broth, water, and bay leaf and bring to a boil. Then reduce the heat and simmer for 15 minutes to meld the flavors.

3. Before serving, add the lemon juice and remove the bay leaf. Season with pepper and additional salt if needed.

Cooking tip: Buy a prechopped mirepoix mix (carrots, onions, and celery) to make prep even faster.

Variation tip: I try to sneak in greens wherever I can, which means I usually add chopped kale or spinach, or both, to my bowl before pouring the hot soup over it.

Per Serving: Calories: 556; Fat: 25g; Saturated Fat: 6g; Cholesterol: 215mg; Carbohydrates: 8g; Fiber: 2g; Protein: 71g; Sodium: 842mg

Classic Chili

Nut-Free

When making this hearty dish, I usually reach for bison rather than beef because it has fewer calories and less fat but has the exact same flavor profile. If you do choose beef, purchase 92 percent lean or higher. Ground turkey is also a lean option, but it will change the taste slightly.

SERVES 6   *Prep time: 10 minutes / Cook time: 40 minutes*

2 tablespoons extra-virgin olive oil

½ large onion, chopped

1 pound ground bison or lean beef (92/8 or leaner)

½ teaspoon sea salt, plus more as needed

2 garlic cloves, minced

1 large red bell pepper, diced

1 large green bell pepper, diced

2 tablespoons chili powder

1 teaspoon smoked paprika

½ teaspoon ground cumin

1 (28-ounce) can fire-roasted crushed tomatoes

1 (15-ounce) can black, kidney, or pinto beans, drained and rinsed

1 to 2 cups vegetable broth

Sliced avocado and lime for serving (optional)

1. In a large pot, heat the oil over medium-high heat. Add the onion, bison, and salt. Sauté until the bison begins to brown, about 5 minutes.

2. Add the garlic, bell peppers, chili powder, paprika, and cumin and continue to sauté until the vegetables soften and become fragrant, an additional 3 to 5 minutes.

3. Add the tomatoes, beans, and 1 cup of vegetable broth. Bring to a boil, then reduce the heat to low, cover, and simmer for 25 to 30 minutes. Add ½ to 1 cup more broth if you want a looser chili. Taste and see if it needs more salt.

4. Serve with sliced avocado and a squeeze of lime, if desired.

Ingredient tip: Your body absorbs iron best when it's paired with vitamin C. In this recipe you'll get iron from the meat and the vitamin C from both the peppers and tomatoes will help you absorb it.

Per Serving: Calories: 335; Fat: 17g; Saturated Fat: 6g; Cholesterol: 53mg; Carbohydrates: 24g; Fiber: 7.5g; Protein: 21g; Sodium: 814mg

6

Seafood & Vegetarian Meals

Easy Egg Frittata with Sun-Dried Tomato and Artichokes

Vegetarian, Nut-Free

This dish can easily be a breakfast, lunch, or dinner. It pairs well with a really light, simple green salad with a bit of avocado. The sun-dried tomatoes add a delicious depth of flavor. I usually buy the ones sold in a bag, but if you get the tomatoes packed in oil, just drain before chopping. Either will do.

SERVES 4 *Prep time: 10 minutes, plus 5 minutes to stand / Cook time: 20 minutes*

2 tablespoons extra-virgin olive oil, divided

10 large eggs or 2 cups liquid eggs

½ cup diced onion

1 cup canned water-packed artichoke hearts, drained and chopped

½ cup chopped dry-packed sun-dried tomatoes

½ teaspoon sea salt

1. Preheat the oven to 375°F. Coat a 10-inch baking dish with 1 tablespoon of oil.

2. Crack the eggs into a blender and blend on high until they become whipped and frothy, about 1 minute.

3. In a medium saucepan, heat the remaining 1 tablespoon of oil over medium heat. Add the onion, artichoke hearts, sun-dried tomatoes, and salt. Sauté until the onion becomes translucent and the vegetables soften, 3 to 4 minutes.

4. Transfer the vegetables to the prepared baking dish and pour the eggs over.

5. Bake until the edges brown and egg is set, about 15 minutes.

6. Let stand an additional 5 minutes to complete cooking and begin to cool before slicing and serving.

Cooking tip: If you have an ovenproof skillet, save time and use one pan for this recipe.

Per Serving: Calories: 289; Fat: 19g; Saturated Fat: 5g; Cholesterol: 465mg; Carbohydrates: 11g; Fiber: 2g; Protein: 18g; Sodium: 666mg

Southwestern Black Bean Quinoa Bowl

Vegan, Nut-Free

Warm bowls like this make comforting, all-in-one lunches or dinners in the cooler months. And with your quinoa prepped ahead of time, the meal comes together so quickly. Add a dollop of Edamame Guacamole (page 55) to each bowl for an extra boost of flavor, color, and nutrition.

SERVES 4   *Prep time: 10 minutes / Cook time: 20 minutes*

2 tablespoons extra-virgin olive oil, divided

½ onion, diced

2 garlic cloves, minced

1 jalapeño pepper (optional), seeded and thinly sliced

2 teaspoons Southwestern or Mexican seasoning

1 (15-ounce) can black beans, drained and rinsed

3 medium tomatoes, such as Roma or plum, diced

1 (16-ounce) package coleslaw mix

¼ cup chopped fresh cilantro

1 orange, peeled and chopped

1 tablespoon freshly squeezed lime juice

½ teaspoon sea salt

2 cups cooked quinoa, warmed

1. In a large skillet, heat 1 tablespoon of oil over medium heat. Add the onion, garlic, jalapeño pepper (if using), and seasoning, and sauté until the onion softens, 3 to 5 minutes.

2. Add the beans and tomatoes and simmer over low heat until everything is softened, 10 to 15 minutes.

3. Meanwhile, in a large bowl, combine the coleslaw mix, cilantro, orange, lime juice, remaining 1 tablespoon of oil, and the salt.

4. To serve, divide the warmed quinoa into bowls and top with the black bean mixture. Top the beans with the slaw.

Ingredient tip: Quinoa is gluten-free and high in protein and fiber, making it a great option when you're craving a comforting grain like rice or pasta.

Storage tip: The entire bowl (combined) will keep for 3 to 4 days in your refrigerator. You can keep the slaw separate if you want to keep it crunchy before reheating the quinoa and beans, or keep all the ingredients together and eat it cold or warmed.

Per Serving: Calories: 335; Fat: 9g; Saturated Fat: 1.5g; Cholesterol: 0mg; Carbohydrates: 52g; Fiber: 13g; Protein: 13g; Sodium: 500mg

Pesto Zoodles with Crunchy Chickpeas

Vegan

Thick, rich pesto meets fresh, light zucchini for a serious comfort dish made healthy. Add sun-dried tomatoes for a pop of color, and top with crunchy chickpeas for added texture, fiber, and protein. You'll love this satisfying meal.

SERVES 4   *Prep time: 15 minutes / Cook time: 5 minutes*

4 medium to large zucchini, spiralized, or 2 (10-ounce) packages zucchini noodles

1 teaspoon sea salt

⅓ cup Spinach-Walnut Pesto (page 137)

1 teaspoon extra-virgin olive oil

1 cup drained oil-packed sun-dried tomatoes, chopped

1 tablespoon freshly squeezed lemon juice

1 cup Herby Roasted Chickpeas (page 58)

1. Line a baking sheet or cutting board with paper towels and lay out the spiralized zucchini. Sprinkle with the salt and let sit for 10 to 15 minutes to allow the zucchini to release some water.

2. Meanwhile, in a small saucepan on the stove or in a microwave-safe bowl in the microwave, warm the pesto, adding hot water if needed to thin it slightly.

3. In a large nonstick skillet, heat the oil over medium-high heat. Add the zucchini and cook for 1 to 2 minutes. Add the pesto, sun-dried tomatoes, and lemon juice, tossing to coat evenly. Sauté until everything is warm and your zucchini is cooked to your preferred texture, an additional 1 to 2 minutes.

4. Divide into bowls and top with crispy chickpeas.

Ingredient tip: You can fairly easily find zucchini already spiralized in the store, so keep your eyes peeled.

Cooking tip: Don't skip step 1. Zucchini is 95 percent water and salting it to release some of the liquid will help prevent very watery noodles when you heat them.

Per Serving: Calories: 243; Fat: 15g; Saturated Fat: 2g; Cholesterol: 0mg; Carbohydrates: 24g; Fiber: 7g; Protein: 8g; Sodium: 777mg

Greek Goulash with Crispy Baked Tofu

Vegan, Nut-Free

My grandmother is Greek, so I grew up with a few classic Greek dishes. One of my favorites was always our version of goulash. Traditional goulash has meat and vegetables, but our family just used veggies. This recipe bakes slowly over a few hours, so plan to make this on a day you are home for a while.

SERVES 4   *Prep time: 15 minutes / Cook time: 3 to 4 hours*

1 medium eggplant, cut into 2-inch pieces

3 medium zucchini, cut into 2-inch pieces

1 onion, sliced

1 head celery, chopped (including leafy tops, if you have them)

1 (15-ounce) can crushed tomatoes

3 tablespoons extra-virgin olive oil

½ teaspoon sea salt

5 to 7 baby red potatoes, quartered

1 pound green beans

½ cup chopped fresh parsley

Crispy Tofu (page 140) or 4 ounces cooked protein of your choice

1. Preheat the oven to 325°F.
2. In a large roasting pan, combine the eggplant, zucchini, onion, celery (including the tops), and tomatoes and toss with the oil and salt.
3. Roast for 1½ hours, stirring every 20 to 30 minutes.
4. At 1½ hours, add the potatoes and green beans. Return the pan to the oven and continue roasting until all the vegetables are soft and tender, another 1½ to 2½ hours (a total of 3 to 4 hours), depending on the size of the vegetables.
5. Remove from the oven, add the fresh parsley, and serve with a side of baked tofu.

Cooking tip: Cut all the vegetables to similar sizes to ensure even cooking time.

Storage tip: You'll almost definitely have leftovers. Keep covered in the refrigerator for 3 to 4 days. It may not seem like it, but this dish pairs perfectly with eggs.

Per Serving: Calories: 488; Fat: 20g; Saturated Fat: 3g; Cholesterol: 0mg; Carbohydrates: 61g; Fiber: 17g; Protein: 21g; Sodium: 933mg

Moroccan Spiced Lentils with Roasted Cauliflower

Vegan

This dish combines a Moroccan spice blend with black lentils, carrots, golden raisins, cauliflower, and slivered almonds to make a warm and sumptuous meal reminiscent of the souks of Marrakech.

SERVES 4 *Prep time: 10 minutes / Cook time: 40 minutes*

1 head cauliflower, chopped

2 tablespoons coconut oil, divided

1 teaspoon ground turmeric

½ teaspoon ground coriander

1 teaspoon ground cumin

1 teaspoon ground ginger

1 teaspoon sea salt

1 cup diced onion

1 cup black lentils

1 pint cherry tomatoes, halved

½ cup vegetable broth

4 cups packed baby spinach

½ cup slivered almonds, toasted

½ cup golden raisins

Freshly squeezed lemon juice and parsley, for serving (optional)

1. Preheat the oven to 400°F.

2. In a bowl, toss together the cauliflower, 1 tablespoon of oil, and the turmeric. Spread it on a large sheet pan and roast until it's soft and browned, about 40 minutes, stirring once or twice.

3. Meanwhile, in a small bowl, combine the coriander, cumin, ginger, and salt. In a medium saucepan, heat the remaining 1 tablespoon of oil over medium heat. Add the onion and sauté until softened and translucent, 2 to 3 minutes. Add the lentils and spice mixture, and toast for 1 minute. Add the tomatoes and broth, and simmer until the lentils have softened, about 20 minutes.

4. When the cauliflower is done, transfer it to a large bowl. Add the spinach, almonds, and raisins and toss.

5. Place the lentil mixture in the bottom of a shallow dish with cauliflower mixture served on top. Add a squeeze of lemon juice and parsley, if desired.

Per Serving: Calories: 454; Fat: 15g; Saturated Fat: 6.5g; Cholesterol: 0mg; Carbohydrates: 66g; Fiber: 18g; Protein: 22g; Sodium: 750mg

Buddha Bowls

Vegan, Nut-Free

The basic premise of building a wholesome veggie bowl is to divide your bowl into thirds: For the first third, use a starch, grain, or salad greens; for the second, add any combination of vegetables; and for the third, include a protein. Add fat on top, like avocado, nuts, and/or seeds, then drizzle with a sauce or dressing, and voilà! A satisfying meal any time of day.

SERVES 4 *Prep time: 10 minutes / Cook time: 30 minutes*

4 cups roughly chopped broccoli

2 medium sweet potatoes, cubed

2 tablespoons extra-virgin olive oil

4 cups chopped crisp greens, such as romaine

4 cups cooked tofu or lean protein of your choice (see Tip)

2 avocados, sliced

Creamy Lemon-Tahini Dressing (page 132) or ½ cup sauce/dressing of choice

1. Preheat the oven to 375°F.

2. On a sheet pan, toss the broccoli and sweet potatoes with the oil. Roast until tender, 25 to 30 minutes.

3. Divide the greens among four bowls. Add the warm roasted broccoli on one side and warmed sweet potato on the other. On the final third, add the protein.

4. Top each bowl with sliced avocado, then drizzle each bowl with dressing and serve.

Ingredient tip: This recipe is delicious with Crispy Tofu (page 140), Garlicky Green Turkey Meatballs (page 97), or the shrimp from Seared Shrimp with Crunchy Broccoli Slaw (page 87).

Variation tip: Try arugula in place of romaine, and any roasted vegetable, such as cauliflower or Brussels sprouts. For extra crunch, top with a tablespoon or two of slivered almonds, chopped walnuts, or sunflower seeds. Get creative with your bowl and your flavors.

Per Serving: Calories: 624; Fat: 32g; Saturated Fat: 5g; Cholesterol: 119mg; Carbohydrates: 35g; Fiber: 13g; Protein: 53g; Sodium: 854mg

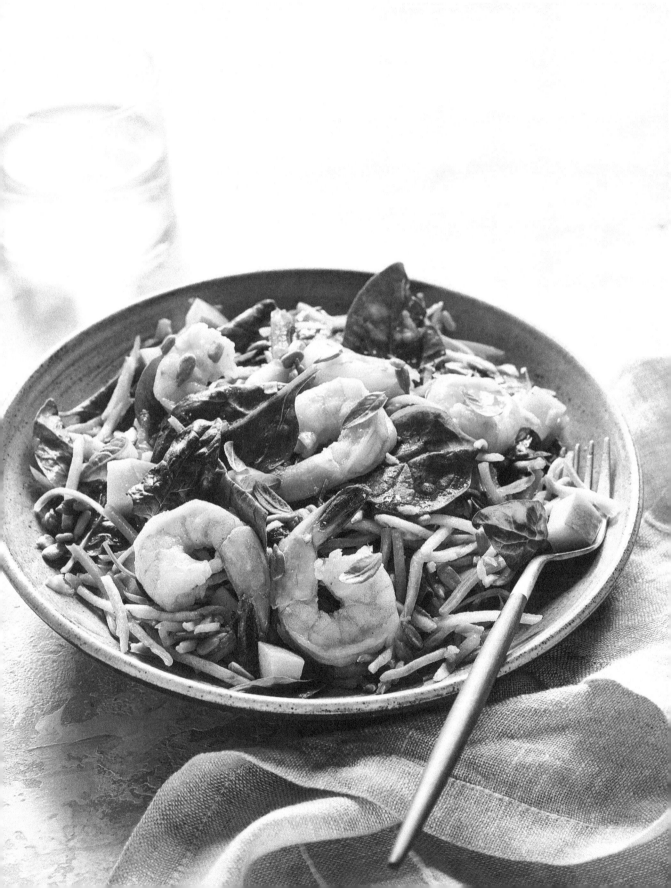

Seared Shrimp with Crunchy Broccoli Slaw

Fast, Nut-Free

Warm shrimp meets cool, crunchy broccoli slaw for a super-fast and satisfying weeknight dish. Here I use a bag of broccoli slaw purchased from the grocery store. I like adding baby spinach for volume, apple for tartness, basil for fresh flavor, and sunflower seeds for crunch, though any of that could easily be omitted—use what you have on hand.

SERVES 4   *Prep time: 10 minutes / Cook time: 10 minutes*

2 (12- to 16-ounce) packages broccoli slaw

2 Granny Smith apples, diced

2 (8-ounce) bags baby spinach

¼ cup chopped fresh basil, plus more (optional) for garnish

1 teaspoon freshly ground black pepper

3 to 4 tablespoons Champagne Vinaigrette (page 131)

2 tablespoons extra-virgin olive oil

1 pound peeled and deveined medium shrimp

¼ cup salted roasted sunflower seeds

1. In a large bowl, combine the broccoli slaw, apples, spinach, and basil. Add the pepper and vinaigrette and toss to coat. Set aside.

2. In a large skillet, heat the oil over medium-high heat. Add the shrimp and sear, flipping once and cooking until the shrimp turn pink and opaque, about 5 minutes.

3. Divide the salad into bowls. Sprinkle with the sunflower seeds and top with shrimp. Garnish with more fresh basil, if desired.

Ingredient tip: Stock your freezer with raw shrimp. On busy weeknights you can pull out as many as you plan to eat and throw together a fast weeknight meal. Before cooking, quick-thaw the shrimp by running cool water over them.

Per Serving: Calories: 346; Fat: 15g; Saturated Fat: 2g; Cholesterol: 172mg; Carbohydrates: 25g; Fiber: 8g; Protein: 28g; Sodium: 648mg

Roasted Tomatoes with Shrimp

Nut-Free

The roasted tomatoes in this dish soften and burst, creating a bright, fresh, saucy consistency. Serve it over roasted spaghetti squash—either roast it on the same night (just plan ahead, as it will take considerably longer than the shrimp) or reheat it from your meal prep day.

SERVES 4   *Prep time: 10 minutes / Cook time: 20 minutes*

2 cups cherry tomatoes

2 tablespoons extra-virgin olive oil, divided

2 garlic cloves, put through a press or minced

2 tablespoons capers

1 pound peeled and deveined medium shrimp

½ teaspoon sea salt

½ cup chopped fresh parsley

2 tablespoons freshly squeezed lemon juice

Freshly ground black pepper

Easy Roasted Spaghetti Squash (page 138), reheated if necessary

Nutritional yeast, for garnish (optional)

1. Preheat the oven to 425°F.

2. In a large baking dish, toss the cherry tomatoes with 1 tablespoon of oil, the garlic, and capers. Roast for 10 minutes.

3. Meanwhile, in a large bowl, toss together the shrimp, salt, parsley, lemon juice, pepper, and the remaining 1 tablespoon of oil.

4. Remove the tomatoes from the oven and stir in the shrimp. Return to the oven until the shrimp are cooked, an additional 10 minutes.

5. Serve immediately in bowls over warm, roasted spaghetti squash. Sprinkle with nutritional yeast, if desired.

Ingredient tip: Nutritional yeast is a wonderful replacement for cheese. It's loaded with vitamins and other nutrients and imparts a cheesy taste similar to Parmesan. Feel free to sprinkle liberally on top of this dish.

Per Serving: Calories: 493; Fat: 27g; Saturated Fat: 4g; Cholesterol: 123mg; Carbohydrates: 53g; Fiber: 10g; Protein: 17g; Sodium: 1,353mg

Weeknight Salmon Stir-Fry

Fast, Nut-Free

Salmon is a great protein option because it is loaded with impressive nutrients, including omega-3 fats and B vitamins, and is so versatile, quick, and easy to make. In fact, it's so quick, this is a good recipe for a weeknight, and my guess is that it will start to work into your regular rotation.

SERVES 4   *Prep time: 10 minutes / Cook time: 20 minutes*

1 tablespoon coconut oil, divided

1½ pounds salmon, skin removed, cut into 1-inch pieces

3 tablespoons tamari

2 tablespoons rice vinegar

2 tablespoons grated fresh ginger

4 garlic cloves, put through a press or minced

2 teaspoons honey

1 large broccoli stalk, chopped

2 red bell peppers, sliced

1 onion, thinly sliced

10 ounces sugar snap peas

2 (8-ounce) cans sliced water chestnuts (optional), drained

1. In a large skillet, heat ½ tablespoon of oil over medium-high heat. Add the salmon, flipping once or twice and cooking until it becomes firm to the touch and is browned on the edges, about 5 minutes.

2. Meanwhile, in a small bowl, combine the tamari, vinegar, ginger, garlic, and honey.

3. Remove the salmon from the pan and set aside.

4. In the same skillet (wiped clean if necessary), add the remaining ½ tablespoon of oil, the broccoli, bell peppers, onion, peas, and water chestnuts (if using). Sauté the mixture over medium heat until the vegetables start to become tender but still remain slightly crisp, about 10 minutes.

5. Pour the tamari sauce over the vegetables and return the salmon to the pan as well. Gently toss and let the sauce simmer an additional 1 to 2 minutes, coating everything.

6. Divide among four plates and serve.

Ingredient tip: If you don't like the idea of cutting raw salmon, feel free to buy and cook 4 individual 6-ounce pieces (or 1 large piece) and serve on top of vegetables. Try it topped with sriracha, red pepper flakes, and a shake of sesame seeds.

Per Serving: Calories: 340; Fat: 13g; Saturated Fat: 4.5g; Cholesterol: 80mg; Carbohydrates: 20g; Fiber: 5.5g; Protein: 35g; Sodium: 838mg

Foil Pack Salmon with Lemon Asparagus and Dairy-Free Tzatziki

Fast, Nut-Free

I think my mom eats salmon at least twice a week, and I honestly can't blame her. It's so simple to prepare (for one or four people!) and so delicious. It's also packed with omega-3 fatty acids, as well as protein and B vitamins. Cooking in foil packs makes cleanup a breeze. Serve this meal alongside a simple salad of greens tossed with olive oil and lemon.

SERVES 4 *Prep time: 10 minutes / Cook time: 10 minutes*

2 bunches asparagus (about 40 spears), ends trimmed

4 (6-ounce) skin-on salmon fillets

2 tablespoons extra-virgin olive oil

1 teaspoon sea salt

1 teaspoon freshly ground black pepper

1 lemon, thinly sliced

¼ cup Dairy-Free Tzatziki (page 133)

1. Preheat a grill to high heat.
2. While the grill heats, lay out 4 pieces of aluminum foil flat, making sure they're large enough to wrap around the salmon and asparagus.
3. Arrange the trimmed asparagus in the center of each piece of foil and place a salmon fillet on top. Drizzle with the oil and sprinkle with salt and pepper. Lay 2 or 3 lemon slices on top of the salmon.
4. Wrap the foil around the fish and vegetables.
5. Place the foil packs on the grill and cook until the salmon is cooked through and the asparagus is tender, about 10 minutes.
6. Serve with a dollop of tzatziki on top of the salmon.

Cooking tip: You can do this entire recipe in the oven. Bake the fish packets at 375°F for 12 to 15 minutes and swap out the foil for parchment if you prefer.

Per Serving: Calories: 380; Fat: 21g; Saturated Fat: 3g; Cholesterol: 109mg; Carbohydrates: 5g; Fiber: 2.5g; Protein: 41g; Sodium: 791mg

Baked Lemon White Fish with Asparagus, Tomatoes, and Kalamata Olives

Nut-Free

The lemon and olives in this dish pack in the flavor and they pair nicely with a light, flaky white fish, such as haddock or cod. This dish tastes bright and fresh, and works well on its own or served with some quinoa.

SERVES 4 *Prep time: 15 minutes / Cook time: 25 to 30 minutes*

1 bunch asparagus, ends trimmed, spears cut into thirds

1 pint cherry tomatoes

⅓ cup pitted Kalamata olives

1 shallot, chopped

3 tablespoons extra-virgin olive oil, divided

1 teaspoon sea salt, divided

Olive oil cooking spray

1½ to 2 pounds haddock or cod fillets, or other thick, flaky white fish

½ teaspoon freshly ground black pepper

1 lemon, half sliced and half left whole for squeezing

1. Preheat the oven to 400°F.

2. In a medium bowl, combine the asparagus, tomatoes, olives, and shallot. Toss with 2 tablespoons of oil and ½ teaspoon of salt.

3. Coat the bottom of a large baking dish with cooking spray and place the fish in the center. Drizzle the fish with the remaining 1 tablespoon of oil and sprinkle with the pepper and the remaining ½ teaspoon of salt.

4. Arrange the vegetables around the fish (it's okay for them to be touching and overlapping with little space in the pan). Arrange the lemon slices on top of the fish and squeeze the juice from the remaining half over the entire dish.

5. Bake until the fish is firm and flakes easily, 25 to 30 minutes.

Per Serving: Calories: 303; Fat: 15g; Saturated Fat: 1.5g; Cholesterol: 107mg; Carbohydrates: 8g; Fiber: 2.5g; Protein: 35g; Sodium: 636mg

Hometown Crab Cakes

Crab cakes were a staple growing up in our home in Baltimore. To this day, my mom will make them as a fun dinner for us when we come home for a visit. These crab cakes are baked, not pan-fried, so there is no added oil in the cooking. Serve with a roasted green vegetable of your choice or a simple salad.

SERVES 4   *Prep time: 30 minutes / Cook time: 15 minutes*

2 large eggs

⅓ cup avocado oil mayonnaise

¼ cup minced celery

2 tablespoons freshly squeezed lemon juice

2 tablespoons Old Bay seasoning

2 teaspoons Worcestershire sauce

½ cup gluten-free panko or bread crumbs, toasted

¼ cup almond flour

2 pounds fresh jumbo lump crabmeat

Olive oil cooking spray

Lemon wedges, for serving

1. In a medium bowl, whisk together the eggs, mayonnaise, celery, lemon juice, Old Bay, and Worcestershire sauce. Fold in the panko and almond flour. Add the crab and toss gently, making sure the ingredients are mixed together. Refrigerate for 20 minutes.

2. Meanwhile, preheat the oven to 450°F. Coat a baking sheet with cooking spray.

3. Divide the mixture into 4 equal patties, about 1 inch thick. Place on the baking sheet and bake until the cakes are browned on the edges, 12 to 15 minutes.

4. Serve with lemon wedges.

Per Serving: Calories: 462; Fat: 23g; Saturated Fat: 3g; Cholesterol: 273mg; Carbohydrates: 12g; Fiber: 1g; Protein: 54g; Sodium: 1,059mg

Coconut Thai Curry Mussels

Fast

Don't let mussels intimidate you. With this recipe, I'll walk you through how to clean and prep them. You might be surprised at how simple it really is to prepare these delicious, healthy shellfish. The other ingredients are simple, with big, fulsome flavors. Because this recipe is on the lighter side, serve with a side salad or some roasted asparagus and fingerling potatoes.

SERVES 4   *Prep time: 15 minutes / Cook time: 10 minutes*

2 pounds live mussels

2 tablespoons coconut oil

1 onion, chopped

2 tablespoons minced fresh ginger

4 garlic cloves, minced

2 tablespoons Thai red curry paste

1 (13-ounce) can light coconut milk

1 cup unsweetened almond milk

1 tablespoon honey

1 cup chopped fresh basil

1 (8- to 10-ounce) bag baby spinach

1 lime, halved

1. Clean and prepare the mussels by placing them in a colander and rinsing with water. Use a sponge or scrub brush to wipe away any debris or sand. Using a paring knife or your fingers, gently pull out any threads protruding from the side of the mussel; this is called the beard. If any shells are open, tap them on the counter to see if they close. If they don't, discard them.

2. In a large pot, heat the oil over medium-high heat. Add the onion, ginger, and garlic and sauté 3 to 4 minutes. Add the curry paste and cook for 1 minute to meld the flavors. Add the coconut milk, almond milk, and honey. Bring to a boil and cook for 2 to 3 minutes.

3. Add the mussels, cover, and cook over medium heat until most or all of the shells have opened, about 5 minutes. Discard any mussels that did not open. Stir in the basil and baby spinach and squeeze in the lime.

4. Divide the mussels and sauce among four bowls and serve.

Variation tip: Add clams, shrimp, or haddock to this dish to make it a full-on fish stew.

Per Serving: Calories: 316; Fat: 16g; Saturated Fat: 11g; Cholesterol: 40mg; Carbohydrates: 21g; Fiber: 3g; Protein: 21g; Sodium: 1,269mg

7

Poultry

Golden Roasted Chicken and White Beans

Nut-Free

I am a big fan of cooking with chicken thighs. The meat is rich, packed with flavor, and typically doesn't dry out as quickly as a chicken breast. Here I'm having you buy skin-on thighs, which means there will be a bit more fat, but the flavor is worth it. However, if that's a concern, you can definitely use skinless thighs.

SERVES 4   *Prep time: 10 minutes / Cook time: 40 minutes*

1 (15-ounce) can cannellini beans, drained and rinsed

1 pint cherry tomatoes

4 garlic cloves, minced

2 cups cubed (1 to 2 inches) butternut squash

1 teaspoon sea salt, divided

4 or 5 thyme sprigs (optional)

2 tablespoons extra-virgin olive oil, divided

8 bone-in, skin-on chicken thighs (about 3 pounds)

½ teaspoon freshly ground black pepper

¼ cup chicken stock

1. Preheat the oven to 425°F.

2. In a large baking dish (a 9-by-13-inch one works well), combine the beans, tomatoes, garlic, squash, ½ teaspoon of salt, the thyme (if using), and 1 tablespoon of oil and toss to coat.

3. Sprinkle the chicken with the pepper and remaining ½ teaspoon of salt and drizzle with the remaining 1 tablespoon of oil. Nestle the chicken into the bean and vegetable mixture. Pour the chicken stock around the entire mixture, which helps keep everything juicy.

4. Roast until the chicken is golden and has reached an internal temperature of 165°F, about 40 minutes.

Per Serving: Calories: 632; Fat: 37g; Saturated Fat: 9g; Cholesterol: 270mg; Carbohydrates: 27g; Fiber: 7g; Protein: 51g; Sodium: 861mg

Garlicky Green Turkey Meatballs

Nut-Free

Meatballs are such a great item to keep on hand in both your refrigerator and freezer. They are so simple to reheat and so versatile. While you can serve them with a classic marinara sauce, pesto is a delicious alternative. Make it a meal by adding them to roasted spaghetti squash, sautéed zucchini noodles, or even to the top of a salad.

SERVES 4   *Prep time: 15 minutes / Cook time: 25 minutes*

Olive oil cooking spray

1 cup frozen chopped spinach, thawed and drained

1 large egg

¼ cup chopped fresh basil

¼ cup chopped fresh parsley

2 garlic cloves, minced

1 teaspoon onion salt

1 tablespoon extra-virgin olive oil

1 pound ground turkey

1. Preheat the oven to 400°F. Coat a sheet pan with cooking spray.
2. To squeeze the spinach dry, wrap it in paper towels and squeeze with your hands.
3. In a large bowl, beat the egg, then add the spinach, basil, parsley, garlic, onion salt, and oil and stir to combine.
4. Using a spoon, break up the turkey, then add to the spinach mixture and combine well. Shape the mixture into 12 meatballs about 2 inches in diameter. Place them on the sheet pan as you finish.
5. Bake until they reach an internal temperature of 165°F, about 25 minutes, flipping halfway so they brown on all sides. Serve immediately or refrigerate for up to 4 days.

Storage tip: If you're already going through the trouble of making these, it's worth the little bit of extra effort to make a double batch. Cook as directed and then store in a resealable plastic bag or freezer-safe container for up to 3 months in the freezer.

Per Serving (3 meatballs): Calories: 229; Fat: 13g; Saturated Fat: 3g; Cholesterol: 122mg; Carbohydrates: 2.5g; Fiber: 1.5g; Protein: 26g; Sodium: 563mg

Roasted Veggie and Chicken Sausage One-Pan Meal

Nut-Free

Not only is cleaning up after this dinner a breeze thanks to the simplicity of cooking in one pan, but it also checks all the major nutrition boxes, providing you with protein, fiber-rich vegetables, and smart carbohydrates. Serve over a bed of greens and top with one-third of an avocado and a squeeze of lime or 2 tablespoons of toasted nuts to add healthy fat and elevate your meal.

SERVES 4   *Prep time: 10 minutes / Cook time: 30 minutes*

Olive oil cooking spray

1 (12-ounce) package fully cooked chicken sausages (about 4), sliced

2 medium sweet potatoes, peeled and cubed

1 large broccoli stalk, chopped

1 red onion, sliced

2 tablespoons extra-virgin olive oil

½ teaspoon sea salt

½ teaspoon freshly ground black pepper

1. Preheat the oven to 400°F. Coat a large sheet pan with cooking spray.

2. Arrange the sausage, sweet potato, broccoli, and onion on the pan. Drizzle with the oil and sprinkle with the salt and pepper.

3. Roast for 15 minutes. Stir with a spatula and bake until the sweet potatoes are fork-tender and veggies are lightly browned, additional 10 to 15 minutes. Serve hot.

Ingredient tip: Not all chicken sausage is made equal. I like the brand Bilinski's, which makes both organic and conventional sausages, and uses minimally processed ingredients.

Variation tip: You can swap out broccoli for another cruciferous vegetable, such as cauliflower, bok choy, Brussels sprouts, or whatever you have on hand!

Per Serving: Calories: 255; Fat: 10g; Saturated Fat: 1.5g; Cholesterol: 69mg; Carbohydrates: 22g; Fiber: 4g; Protein: 19g; Sodium: 968mg

Sheet Pan Chicken Fajitas

Nut-Free

Weeknights are a blur in my family and I am sure many of you can relate. Hence my love of sheet pan meals. One pan to clean, one simple cooking time—it doesn't get easier. Try assembling these in a burrito-style bowl with salsa, avocado, chopped lettuce, and riced cauliflower. You can also put them into romaine leaves to make "taco shells."

SERVES 4   *Prep time: 10 minutes / Cook time: 30 minutes*

3 bell peppers (any color), sliced

1 red onion, sliced

2 to 4 tablespoons taco seasoning, divided

2 tablespoons extra-virgin olive oil, divided

1 pound boneless, skinless chicken breasts

1 (10-ounce) bag riced cauliflower

2 avocados

Juice of 1 lime

1 teaspoon sea salt

1. Preheat the oven to 425°F.

2. Toss the bell peppers and onion directly on a large sheet pan with 1 tablespoon of taco seasoning and 1 tablespoon of oil. Place the chicken breasts on top of the vegetables. Sprinkle them with the remaining 1 tablespoon of oil and more taco seasoning to taste.

3. Roast until chicken has reached an internal temperature of 165°F, about 30 minutes.

4. Meanwhile, prepare the riced cauliflower according to the package directions. In a bowl, mash the avocados with the lime juice and salt.

5. Let the chicken rest for 5 minutes and then slice. Divide into bowls with toppings of choice, such as salsa.

Ingredient tip: If possible, look for an organic taco seasoning that is free of artificial flavors and preservatives.

Cooking tip: I like to keep the chicken breasts whole so that they stay juicy during cooking. If you prefer, you can slice the chicken before cooking, paying close attention to cooking time as the chicken may cook faster.

Per Serving: Calories: 360; Fat: 21g; Saturated Fat: 3g; Cholesterol: 84mg; Carbohydrates: 17g; Fiber: 8.5g; Protein: 29g; Sodium: 823mg

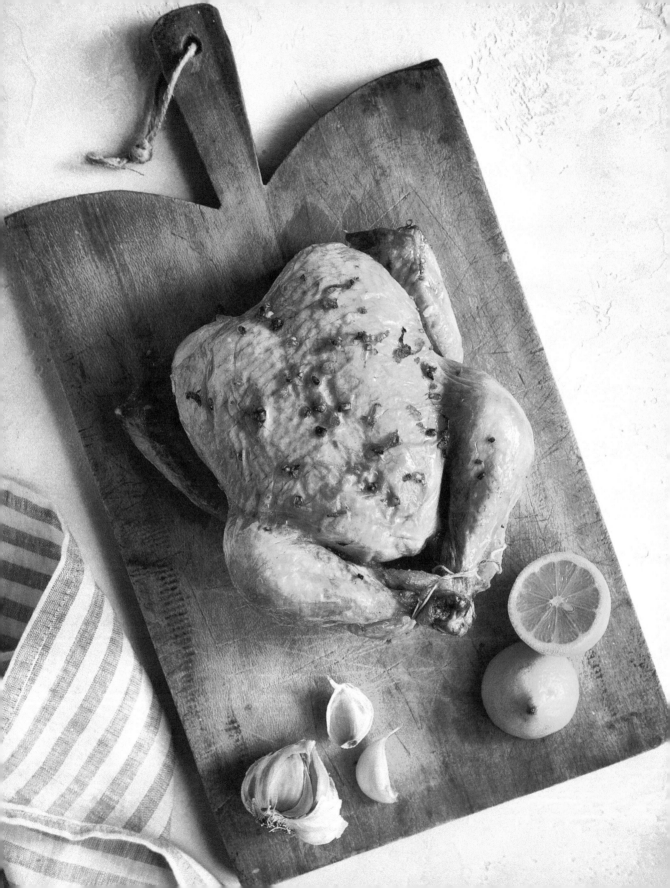

Sunday Lemon-Garlic Roast Chicken

Nut-Free

A roast chicken on a weekend is easy and delicious and should yield lots of leftovers to include in meals like Buddha Bowls (page 85). Serve this chicken alongside roasted cauliflower, broccoli, and carrots, which you can toss with some extra-virgin olive oil and roast for the last 30 minutes of the chicken's cook time.

SERVES 4 (OR 2 WITH LEFTOVERS)
Prep time: 5 minutes/ Cook time: 1 hour 15 minutes to 1 hour 30 minutes

1 (5-pound) whole chicken

2 tablespoons extra-virgin olive oil

4 garlic cloves, minced

Grated zest and juice of 2 lemons

2 teaspoons sea salt

2 teaspoons freshly ground black pepper

1. Preheat the oven to 400°F.

2. Remove any giblets from inside the chicken and discard.

3. Set the chicken breast-side up in a shallow roasting pan and pat it dry with a paper towel.

4. In a small bowl, combine the oil, garlic, lemon zest, lemon juice, salt, and pepper. Rub the mixture all over the outside of the chicken.

5. Roast the chicken uncovered for 45 minutes and then baste with the pan juices. Return to the oven and continue to roast, checking every 15 minutes until the internal temperature reaches 165°F.

6. Let the chicken rest for 5 to 10 minutes before carving and serving.

Variation tip: Try adding 1 tablespoon each of various herbs, such as dried thyme, rosemary, or herbes de Provence, to the chicken. You can also stuff the cavity with lemon, garlic, and fresh herbs to infuse it with even more flavor.

Per Serving: Calories: 379; Fat: 17g; Saturated Fat: 4g; Cholesterol: 163mg; Carbohydrates: 0g; Fiber: 0g; Protein: 53g; Sodium: 739mg

Bruschetta Chicken with Sautéed Spinach and Quinoa

Nut-Free

A take-off on Italy's favorite antipasto, this dish is a showstopper, especially in the summer when tomatoes are in season and basil is fragrant. But don't let the season stop you; this hearty and delicious meal is satisfying all year round.

SERVES 4   *Prep time: 15 minutes / Cook time: 1 hour*

2 cups water

1 cup quinoa, rinsed

6 large Roma (plum) tomatoes, chopped

½ to 1 cup chopped fresh basil, plus more for garnish

4 garlic cloves, put through a press or minced

3 tablespoons balsamic vinegar

1 teaspoon sea salt, divided

2 tablespoons extra-virgin olive oil, divided

1 (10-ounce) container baby spinach (keep the spinach in the container)

8 (3-ounce) chicken breast cutlets

Balsamic glaze (optional; see Tip), for drizzling

1. Preheat the oven to 375°F.

2. In a medium saucepan, combine the water and quinoa. Bring to a boil, cover, and cook according to the package directions.

3. Meanwhile, in a medium bowl, combine the tomatoes, basil, garlic, vinegar, ½ teaspoon of salt, and 1 table-spoon of oil.

4. Pour the remaining 1 tablespoon of oil directly into the container of baby spinach and shake to coat. Pour all of the spinach into a 9-by-13-inch baking dish (or a size you have that will fit chicken).

5. Nestle the chicken cutlets on top of and around the spinach and sprinkle with the remaining ½ teaspoon salt. Top the chicken with the tomato mixture and spread to evenly distribute on and around.

6. Cover with foil and bake for 15 minutes. Uncover and bake until the chicken is cooked through but still juicy, an additional 15 to 20 minutes, depending on the thickness of the cutlets.

7. Serve the tomato-topped chicken over cooked quinoa and garnish with fresh basil and a drizzle of balsamic glaze (if using).

Ingredient tip: Balsamic glaze is a reduced-down version of balsamic vinegar used as a finishing garnish. It elevates the flavors of a meal, and once you've tasted it, you'll likely start drizzling it over all your salads and other dishes, too. Look for it in the same area where regular balsamic vinegar is sold. You can also make your own; there are many recipes online.

Per Serving: Calories: 494; Fat: 14g; Saturated Fat: 2g; Cholesterol: 124mg; Carbohydrates: 41g; Fiber: 5g; Protein: 48g; Sodium: 730mg

Grilled Turkey Burgers with Mango and Avocado

Nut-Free

The combination of mango and avocado gives these burgers a tropical flair. I recommend creating a "bun" out of crunchy iceberg lettuce, which is sturdy and allows you to eat with your hands just like a traditional bun. Pair this meal with oven-roasted sweet potato wedges for a super-satisfying dinner.

SERVES 4   *Prep time: 15 minutes, plus 15 minutes to chill / Cook time: 45 minutes*

3 large sweet potatoes, cut into wedges

2 tablespoons extra-virgin olive oil

1 pound ground turkey

1 teaspoon sea salt

½ teaspoon garlic powder or onion powder

12 to 16 large outer leaves of iceberg lettuce

2 avocados, sliced or mashed

1 large mango, thinly sliced

Optional condiments of choice, like avocado oil mayonnaise

1. Preheat the oven to 400°F.

2. Toss the sweet potatoes with the oil and spread on a sheet pan. Roast until tender but crispy on the outside, about 30 minutes, flipping once during baking.

3. Meanwhile, in a large bowl, combine the turkey, salt, and garlic powder and mix well. Form into 4 equal patties. Refrigerate for 15 minutes.

4. Preheat a grill to high heat.

5. Grill the patties until they are browned on both sides and cooked to an internal temperature of 165°F, 4 to 6 minutes per side.

6. Let the patties rest for 5 minutes and then assemble each burger by placing a patty inside 2 or 3 lettuce leaves, topping with avocado, mango, and any condiments. Place another lettuce leaf on top. Serve with sweet potato wedges.

Cooking tip: If you don't have a grill, you can cook these in the oven with your sweet potatoes, for 10 to 15 minutes, or until firm to the touch.

Per Serving: Calories: 480; Fat: 26g; Saturated Fat: 4.5g; Cholesterol: 76mg; Carbohydrates: 40g; Fiber: 9.5g; Protein: 26g; Sodium: 710mg

Chicken Kebabs with Corn on the Cob

Fast, Nut-Free

Prepare this summertime classic with even more ease by buying premade meat and vegetable kebabs at the store. Just opt for ones that have not been marinated. I'm using chicken here, but feel free to swap in shrimp, salmon, steak, or even tofu.

SERVES 4 *Prep time: 10 minutes / Cook time: 10 minutes*

3 bell peppers, any color, cut into 1-inch pieces

1 sweet onion, such as Vidalia, cut into 1-inch wedges

3 or 4 medium zucchini, cut into 1-inch-thick rounds

1½ pounds boneless, skinless chicken breasts, cut into 1-inch chunks

2 tablespoons avocado oil

2 tablespoons balsamic vinegar

2 teaspoons sea salt

4 ears corn, shucked

1 tablespoon extra-virgin olive oil

1. Preheat a grill to high heat. If using wooden skewers, soak them for at least 20 minutes in water.

2. In a large bowl, combine the bell peppers, onion, zucchini, and chicken and toss with the avocado oil, vinegar, and salt.

3. Prepare kebabs by threading the chicken, bell pepper, onion, and zucchini, alternating ingredients. The number of skewers you make will vary depending on skewer size.

4. Reduce the grill heat to medium and set up for two-zone cooking. Grill the kebabs over direct heat, rotating to cook evenly, 10 to 15 minutes.

5. Brush the corn with the olive oil and grill over indirect heat. Once the corn begins to char, remove from the grill, followed by the kebabs once the chicken is cooked through.

Cooking tip: You can skip the skewers altogether and throw all the ingredients into a large grill basket to save time and energy.

Per Serving: Calories: 416; Fat: 12g; Saturated Fat: 2.5g; Cholesterol: 94mg; Carbohydrates: 40g; Fiber: 7g; Protein: 43g; Sodium: 858mg

Chicken Pad Thai

Fast

You won't believe how easy and fast it is to make flavorful pad Thai at home from scratch. With complete control over the ingredients, you can avoid preservatives and unnecessary added sugars found in many prepared sauces, and also keep things low-carb and high-protein. Speaking of low-carb, we're using shirataki noodles, which are made up of water and fiber (from a type of Japanese root vegetable called konjac) and are basically neutral-tasting and calorie-free. While their texture can be a bit chewy, it doesn't matter in a dish that typically uses rice noodles.

SERVES 4   *Prep time: 10 minutes / Cook time: 15 minutes*

3 tablespoons fish sauce

¼ cup tamari

2 tablespoons honey

4 garlic cloves, minced

Juice of 4 limes
(4 to 6 tablespoons)

2 (7-ounce) packages
shirataki noodles

4 tablespoons coconut oil,
divided

2 (8-ounce) boneless,
skinless chicken breasts,
sliced

4 large eggs

2 cups frozen shelled
edamame, thawed

1. In a bowl, whisk together the fish sauce, tamari, honey, garlic, and lime juice. Set the sauce aside.

2. Prepare the noodles according to the package directions (the noodles have a slight smell, but once you rinse them thoroughly that will go away).

3. In a large skillet, heat 2 tablespoons of oil over high heat (the hotter the pan the better). Add the noodles and sauté for 2 minutes. Remove from the pan and set aside.

4. Reduce the heat to medium, add the remaining 2 tablespoons of oil and the chicken, letting it brown on both sides. Once the chicken is cooked through, push to the side of the pan.

5. Add the eggs to the pan and scramble. Push to the side.

6. Add the reserved sauce, the edamame, and noodles to the pan and stir everything together. Bring to a boil and then remove from the heat. Add the bean sprouts and cilantro, and toss until everything is evenly distributed.

2 cups bean sprouts

¾ cup chopped fresh cilantro

¾ cup salted roasted peanuts (optional), roughly chopped

Lime wedges (optional), for serving

7. Serve in bowls. If desired, top with crushed peanuts and serve with a lime for squeezing.

Variation tip: Replace the chicken with pressed firm tofu or shrimp.

Per Serving: Calories: 515; Fat: 24g; Saturated Fat: 13g; Cholesterol: 269mg; Carbohydrates: 29g; Fiber: 8g; Protein: 45g; Sodium: 2,223mg

Dijon Turkey with Roasted Vegetables

Nut-Free

Everyone knows that turkey is great in a sandwich for lunch. And it wouldn't really feel like Thanksgiving without some form of turkey to go with all the fixings. Yet this versatile bird often gets overlooked for a spot in the weeknight dinner rotation. Truth be told, a boneless turkey breast is as easy to cook as a chicken breast, and the Dijon mustard in this recipe brings out the unique flavor of roast turkey.

SERVES 4 *Prep time: 10 minutes / Cook time: 45 minutes*

2 pounds boneless turkey breast halves

1 teaspoon Dijon mustard

1 teaspoon sea salt, divided

2 tablespoons extra-virgin olive oil, divided

2 teaspoons herbes de Provence or 1 teaspoon each dried rosemary and thyme

1 pound Brussels sprouts, halved

4 cups chopped peeled butternut squash

1. Preheat the oven to 425°F.
2. Place the turkey in the center of a large sheet pan.
3. In a small bowl, combine the mustard, ½ teaspoon of salt, 1 tablespoon of oil, and the herbs. Rub the mixture all over the turkey.
4. Roast the turkey for 10 minutes.
5. Meanwhile, in a large bowl, toss the Brussels sprouts and squash with the remaining 1 tablespoon of oil and ½ teaspoon of salt.
6. After the turkey has finished roasting, add the vegetables to the same pan, return to the oven, and roast until the vegetables are tender and the internal temperature of the turkey reads 165°F. Start checking the turkey when it has been in for 40 minutes. If one is done before the other, remove the vegetables or turkey and cover to keep warm.
7. Let the turkey rest for 5 minutes before slicing and serving with the roasted vegetables.

Per Serving: Calories: 391; Fat: 6.5g; Saturated Fat: 1.5g; Cholesterol: 143mg; Carbohydrates: 25g; Fiber: 6.5g; Protein: 59g; Sodium: 820mg

Fried Cauliflower Rice with Chicken Sausage

Fast, Nut-Free

Another fast and flavorful one-pan dish to have in your regular rotation, this meal is a spin-off of the classic fried rice you grew up with. Instead of white rice, you'll use riced cauliflower to keep the carbohydrates and calories low. It also adds a boost of fiber.

SERVES 4   *Prep time: 10 minutes / Cook time: 15 minutes*

1 teaspoon sesame oil

2 tablespoons tamari

2 garlic cloves, minced

1 tablespoon sesame seeds

1 tablespoon coconut oil

8 fully cooked chicken sausages, cut into rounds

1 (10-ounce) bag frozen riced cauliflower

3 cups shredded green cabbage

1 cup shredded carrots

10 ounces snow peas, chopped

1 cup chopped scallions

1 lime, cut into wedges

1. In a small bowl, whisk together the sesame oil, tamari, garlic, and sesame seeds. Set aside.

2. In a large skillet, heat the coconut oil over medium heat. Add the chicken sausages and sauté until the sausages begin to brown. Once browned, add the cauliflower, cabbage, carrots, and 1 tablespoon of the reserved sauce. Toss and cook until everything begins to soften, 5 to 7 minutes.

3. Add the peas and the remaining sauce and continue to cook for another 2 to 3 minutes.

4. To serve, divide among four bowls, top with chopped scallions, and serve with a wedge of lime.

Variation tip: For an extra boost of protein, add two scrambled eggs to the recipe.

Per Serving: Calories: 317; Fat: 11g; Saturated Fat: 4g; Cholesterol: 110mg; Carbohydrates: 22g; Fiber: 6g; Protein: 32g; Sodium: 1,550mg

Buffalo Chicken Stuffed Sweet Potato with Southwest Slaw

Nut-Free

This fun recipe entails stuffing shredded chicken into a baked sweet potato and topping it with cool, crunchy slaw. The chicken is cooked in a fairly neutral stock and then tossed with Buffalo wing sauce after, which means that if you'd like you can set aside some of the shredded chicken to use in other meals. Buy any slaw salad kit you like for the salad and for the sweet potatoes, choose small to medium potatoes to keep portions in check. Bonus: Leftover shredded chicken over salad slaw makes a great lunch!

SERVES 4 (OR 2 WITH LEFTOVERS)   *Prep time: 10 minutes / Cook time: 7 hours*

2 pounds boneless, skinless chicken breasts

1 cup low-sodium chicken stock

4 garlic cloves, peeled but whole

¾ teaspoon sea salt

4 medium sweet potatoes

1 or 2 (10- to 12-ounce) packages coleslaw or Southwest-style chopped salad kits

¼ cup Buffalo wing sauce, or more as needed

1. In a slow cooker, combine the chicken, stock, garlic, and salt. Cook on low for 6 hours. When the chicken is done and has reached an internal temperature of 165°F, shred it in the pot and set on warm until you're ready to eat.

2. Preheat the oven to 375°F.

3. Wash the sweet potatoes and prick with a fork in a few spots. Place them on a baking sheet and bake until fork-tender, 45 minutes to 1 hour. (Alternatively, prick the sweet potatoes and microwave until fork-tender, about 15 minutes.)

4. Meanwhile, prepare the slaw according to the kit directions. Refrigerate until you're ready to eat.

5. If you are serving four people, toss all of the chicken with Buffalo sauce. However, if you are serving two, then toss only half of the shredded chicken with the Buffalo sauce (saving the plain chicken for leftovers).

6. When the potatoes are done, slice them down the middle (being careful of hot steam). Fill each potato with the chicken and top with the slaw. (When serving two, store the remaining sweet potatoes and slaw to be used as leftovers.)

Ingredient tips: Sweet potatoes are packed with vitamins and minerals as well as fiber. While they are considered a starchy carbohydrate, they are still a great food to incorporate into your meals because they are satisfying, help you feel full, and help stabilize your energy levels.

When buying Buffalo wing sauce, look for an option that has low sugar (5 grams or less per serving). You'll find that by looking at the "Added Sugars" line on the Nutrition Facts panel of the jar.

Per Serving: Calories: 516; Fat: 14g; Saturated Fat: 3g; Cholesterol: 184mg; Carbohydrates: 38g; Fiber: 6.5g; Protein: 59g; Sodium: 1,163mg

Beef & Pork

8

Roasted Pork Tenderloin with Red Potatoes and French Beans

Nut-Free

Pork tenderloin is extremely lean, making it one of the healthiest cuts of pork you can buy. Tenderloin is also reasonably priced and one of the less daunting cuts of meat to cook. It will cook quickly, slices easily, and can make great leftovers for lunch. If the weather permits, feel free to cook this on the grill.

SERVES 4   *Prep time: 10 minutes, plus 20 minutes to marinate / Cook time: 30 minutes*

Any Meat Marinade
(page 134)

1½ to 2 pounds pork
tenderloin

½ to 1 pound baby red
potatoes, quartered

1 pound green beans or
haricots verts (French
green beans)

1 tablespoon extra-virgin
olive oil

1 teaspoon sea salt

Olive oil cooking spray

1. Place the marinade and pork in a resealable plastic bag and marinate for at least 20 minutes or up to 4 hours. It's okay to marinate at room temperature for up to 30 minutes, but refrigerate it over that amount of time.

2. Preheat the oven to 400°F.

3. Place the potatoes and green beans on a sheet pan and toss with the oil and salt. Roast for 30 minutes, tossing once or twice during cook time.

4. Meanwhile, coat an ovenproof skillet with cooking spray and heat over medium-high heat. Remove the pork from the marinade and add to the skillet. Sear on one side and then flip, 2 to 3 minutes per side.

5. Transfer the skillet to the oven and roast until the pork reaches an internal temperature of 145°F, about 20 minutes, depending on the thickness of the pork.

6. When done, move the pork to a cutting board and let rest for at least 5 minutes, or until the potatoes and beans are done cooking.

7. Cut the pork into ½-inch-thick slices and serve alongside the potatoes and beans.

Ingredient tip: Haricots verts (aka French green beans) are longer and thinner than regular green beans. I typically keep a bag of them in my freezer. To cook, you can place frozen beans directly into the oven to thaw, about 5 minutes, then toss with oil.

Per Serving: Calories: 323; Fat: 10g; Saturated Fat: 2.5g; Cholesterol: 92mg; Carbohydrates: 22g; Fiber: 4.5g; Protein: 37g; Sodium: 807mg

Burger Bowls

Nut-Free

If you're trying to decide between bison and beef, here is the bottom line: Bison is much leaner than beef, so you'll get less saturated fat, which is better for you. That said, beef is also an okay choice, as long as you choose the leanest option available.

SERVES 4 *Prep time: 20 minutes / Cook time: 10 minutes*

1 pound lean ground beef (92/8 or leaner) or bison

1 teaspoon sea salt

1 tablespoon Dijon mustard

2 heads romaine or lettuce of choice, chopped

1 cup Edamame Guacamole (page 55)

1 pint cherry tomatoes, halved

4 tablespoons Champagne Vinaigrette (optional; page 131)

1. In a large bowl, combine the beef, salt, and mustard. Form into 4 equal patties. Refrigerate for 15 minutes.

2. Preheat a grill or stovetop grill pan. Cook 5 to 10 minutes, depending on desired doneness: an internal temperature of 120° to 125°F for rare, 130° to 135°F for medium rare, 150° to 155°F for medium well, and 160° to 165°F for well-done.

3. To assemble the bowls, make a base of lettuce. Arrange the cherry tomatoes, guacamole, and burger on top. If desired, drizzle with the vinaigrette.

Storage tip: If you're only making this for one or two people, you can freeze the other two burgers, but make sure you halve the other ingredients.

Per Serving: Calories: 361; Fat: 16g; Saturated Fat: 4g; Cholesterol: 76mg; Carbohydrates: 22g; Fiber: 12g; Protein: 34g; Sodium: 792mg

Salsa Verde Shredded Pork and Kale

Nut-Free

This recipe is super easy but also restaurant quality. Here I use boneless pork shoulder, but a tenderloin would also work. Serve it over some simple garlicky braised kale and top with cool red pepper slices, avocado, lime, and cilantro. Plan ahead because this is made in a slow cooker (or use an electric pressure cooker if time is tight).

SERVES 4 (WITH LEFTOVER PORK)   *Prep time: 10 minutes / Cook time: 8 hours*

2½ to 3 pounds boneless pork shoulder or tenderloin

1 (16-ounce) jar salsa verde, plus more (optional) for serving

1 teaspoon sea salt

4 garlic cloves, 2 whole and 2 minced or put through a press

2 teaspoons extra-virgin olive oil

2 (10-ounce) bags chopped kale

1 red bell pepper, sliced

1 avocado, sliced

Cilantro, for garnish

Lime wedges, for squeezing

1. In a slow cooker, combine the pork, salsa verde, salt, and 2 whole garlic cloves. Cook on low for 8 hours. Your meat will be done when it shreds easily with a fork and has reached an internal temperature of 145°F.

2. Once the meat is fully cooked, shred it in the cooker juices and let it sit on warm.

3. In a large skillet, heat the oil over medium-low heat. Add the minced garlic cloves and kale and gently sauté until wilted, about 5 minutes.

4. Divide the kale into four bowls. Using only about three-quarters of the shredded mixture (the rest is for leftovers), top the kale with the pork. Top each bowl equally with the bell pepper, avocado, cilantro, and a squeeze of lime. Serve with additional salsa verde, if desired.

Cooking tip: To make in an electric pressure cooker, combine all the ingredients and set the vent to Sealing. Cook on high pressure for 30 minutes followed by natural release. The entire process should take 50 minutes or so. Once released, shred and serve as directed above.

Per Serving: Calories: 573; Fat: 32g; Saturated Fat: 9.5g; Cholesterol: 121mg; Carbohydrates: 34g; Fiber: 12g; Protein: 43g; Sodium: 1,058mg

Braised Pork Chops with Silky Cabbage and Apple

Nut-Free

When cooked slowly with some olive oil, crunchy cabbage softens into a buttery texture that melts in your mouth. The apples here impart a sweetness and tang that balance perfectly with the salty pork. This dish tastes great alongside cold crisp greens.

SERVES 4   *Prep time: 10 minutes / Cook time: 30 minutes*

2 tablespoons extra-virgin olive oil, divided

4 bone-in center-cut loin pork chops, ½ to 1 inch thick

1 teaspoon sea salt, divided

2 (10–ounce) bags shredded cabbage (or 1 small head cabbage, shredded)

½ onion, thinly sliced

1 Granny Smith apple, diced

1 teaspoon apple cider vinegar

1. Preheat the oven to 350°F.

2. In a large skillet, heat 1 tablespoon of oil over medium-high heat. Season both sides of the pork with ½ teaspoon of salt, add to the pan, and sear until browned, about 3 minutes. Flip and sear the second side.

3. Place the pork on a sheet pan and roast the chops until the internal temperature reaches 145°F, about 15 minutes, depending on the thickness of the chop.

4. Meanwhile, add the remaining 1 tablespoon of oil to the skillet and set over medium-low heat. Add the cabbage, onion, and remaining ½ teaspoon of salt and slowly sauté, stirring occasionally, until the cabbage is tender, about 10 minutes. Stir in the apple and vinegar.

5. To serve, place the cabbage and apple mixture on a plate alongside the pork chop.

Per Serving: Calories: 362; Fat: 19g; Saturated Fat: 3.5g; Cholesterol: 93mg; Carbohydrates: 15g; Fiber: 5g; Protein: 32g; Sodium: 683mg

Sneaky Veggie Bolognese

Nut-Free

I like to maximize the nutrition (and flavor) by sneaking extra vegetables into a Bolognese sauce. To keep carbohydrates low and processed grains at bay, serve yours over Easy Roasted Spaghetti Squash (page 138), lightly sautéed zucchini noodles, or even alongside some basic roasted broccoli.

SERVES 4 *Prep time: 10 minutes / Cook time: 40 minutes*

1 tablespoon extra-virgin olive oil

1 pound lean ground beef (92/8 or leaner) or bison

2 garlic cloves, put through a press

1 red or green bell pepper, diced

2 cups chopped mushrooms

2 carrots, chopped

4 cups baby spinach

Everyday Pasta Sauce (page 135) or 5 cups store-bought pasta sauce (I like Rao's)

Freshly ground black pepper

Sea salt, optional

1. In a large pot, heat the oil over medium-high heat. Add the beef and cook, stirring frequently to break up, until the edges begin to brown, 2 to 3 minutes.

2. Add the garlic, bell pepper, mushrooms, carrots, and spinach. Stir into the meat and continue to sauté over medium-high for 2 to 3 minutes.

3. Add the pasta sauce, bring to a boil, then reduce to low heat and simmer for 30 minutes. Season with black pepper to taste and salt if needed.

Storage tip: Feel free to make a big batch of this, separate into freezer-safe containers of 1-cup portions, and freeze to pull out on busy weeknights for a dinner for one.

Per Serving: Calories: 412; Fat: 22g; Saturated Fat: 5g; Cholesterol: 71mg; Carbohydrates: 23g; Fiber: 8g; Protein: 30g; Sodium: 1,101mg

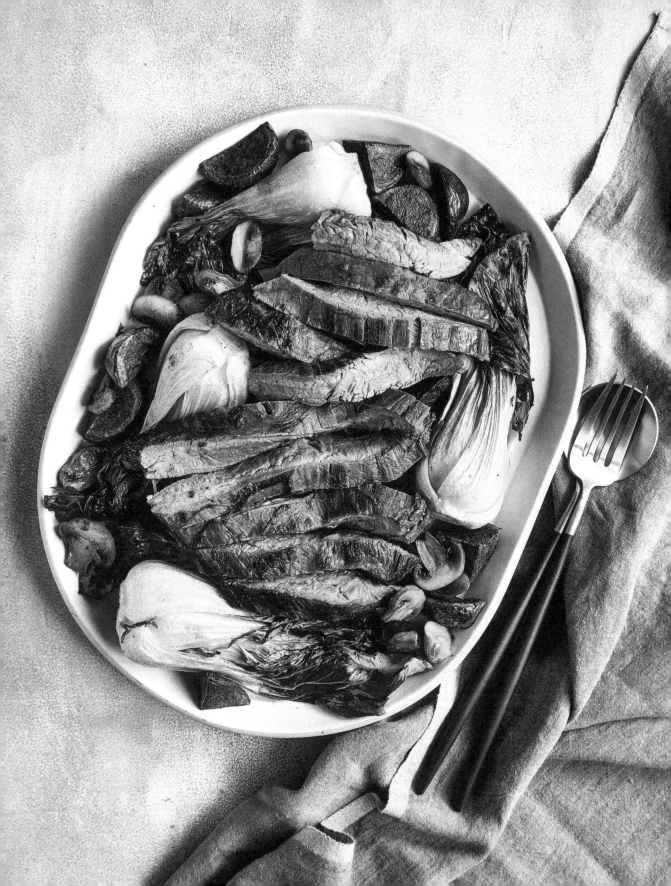

Flank Steak with Mushrooms and Baby Bok Choy

Nut-Free

This is a modern take on the traditional meat and potatoes dinner, and the tamari brings it to another level. Flank steak is a win-win choice; this long and flat cut of beef is typically very lean and very affordable. Flank steak is suitable for everything from grilling to searing to broiling. When serving, slice it thinly against the grain.

SERVES 4   *Prep time: 10 minutes, plus 20 minutes to marinate / Cook time: 30 minutes*

Any Meat Marinade
(page 134)

2 pounds flank steak

1 pound purple potatoes, quartered

1 (8-ounce) container sliced white mushrooms

4 to 8 baby bok choy

2 tablespoons avocado oil, divided

½ teaspoon sea salt

1 tablespoon tamari

1. Place the steak in a large, shallow dish, pour the marinade over, and turn it so the whole steak is covered. Marinate for 20 minutes (or up to 2 hours) in the refrigerator.

2. Preheat the oven to 425°F.

3. In a large bowl, toss together the potatoes, mushrooms, bok choy, 1 tablespoon of oil, the salt, and tamari. Spread on a baking sheet and roast for 20 to 30 minutes, until the potatoes are tender.

4. Meanwhile, heat a large ovenproof skillet over medium-high heat. Add the remaining 1 tablespoon of oil. Once the oil is shimmering hot, sear the steak for 5 minutes (do not move the steak). Flip and sear for another 5 minutes.

5. Transfer the skillet with the steak to the oven and cook until the internal temperature reads at least 130°F for medium-rare, 5 to 10 minutes (the longer time for more well-done beef).

CONTINUED

6. Let the steak rest for 10 minutes before slicing and serving alongside the roasted vegetables.

Ingredient tip: Purple potatoes are higher in antioxidants than other potatoes. That said, feel free to swap for small red or fingerling potatoes if you can't find the purple version.

Cooking tip: This entire meal is fantastic on the grill. Just parboil the potatoes before grilling and use a grill basket for all the vegetables and potatoes.

Per Serving: Calories: 562; Fat: 25g; Saturated Fat: 7.5g; Cholesterol: 145mg; Carbohydrates: 27g; Fiber: 5.5g; Protein: 57g; Sodium: 940mg

Kitchen Sink Stuffed Peppers

Nut-Free

Make this recipe on a night when you've got odds and ends of veggies on hand, such as any leafy greens, onion or garlic, or some diced mushrooms. I only listed basic ingredients here, but don't let that limit you. Get creative! The lamb is a nice change of pace from traditional ground beef here, but you could sub in ground beef or turkey.

SERVES 4 *Prep time: 15 minutes / Cook time: 30 minutes*

Olive oil cooking spray

2 tablespoons extra-virgin olive oil

1 cup diced onion

1 pound ground lamb

1 teaspoon ground cumin

1 teaspoon paprika

½ teaspoon chili powder (optional)

4 cups chopped leafy greens, such as spinach, kale, or collard greens

2 large carrots, diced

4 garlic cloves, minced

4 tablespoons tomato paste

8 bell peppers, any color

1 cup Everyday Pasta Sauce (page 135) or store-bought pasta sauce

½ cup chopped fresh herbs, such as parsley, basil, or cilantro

1. Preheat the oven to 375°F. Coat a glass baking dish with cooking spray.

2. In a medium skillet, heat the oil over medium heat. Add the onion, lamb, cumin, paprika, and chili powder (if using), stirring frequently to break up the meat, until it just begins to brown, 2 to 3 minutes. Add the greens, carrots, and garlic. Cook until the meat is browned and the vegetables are soft, about 10 minutes. Carefully drain off as much fat as you can, stir in the tomato paste, and cook for 1 minute.

3. Meanwhile, carefully slice the stem end off each bell pepper and remove the seeds and ribs.

4. Place the peppers in the baking dish. Spoon the lamb mixture into the peppers and top each pepper with the pasta sauce. Sprinkle with the fresh herbs.

5. Bake until the peppers soften, 10 to 20 minutes.

Per Serving: Calories: 420; Fat: 25g; Saturated Fat: 7.5g; Cholesterol: 75mg; Carbohydrates: 28g; Fiber: 8.5g; Protein: 24g; Sodium: 351mg

Pork Milanese over Balsamic Greens

Fast

Traditional pork Milanese uses a coating of bread crumbs and refined flour, which I swap here for gluten-free panko and almond flour. The panko works right out of the package, but if you toast it before using, it brings a depth of flavor and texture to the coating that is well worth the extra step! I'm serving it over an arugula salad, but feel free to pair it with your favorite vegetable.

SERVES 4   *Prep time: 10 minutes, plus 5 minutes standing / Cook time: 10 minutes*

Olive oil cooking spray

2 cups gluten-free panko

1 teaspoon sea salt, divided

4 large eggs

2 cups almond flour

8 (4-ounce) pork cutlets

1 (10-ounce) bag baby arugula

2 cups cherry tomatoes, halved

2 tablespoons extra-virgin olive oil

1 tablespoon balsamic vinegar

1 lemon (optional)

1. Preheat the oven to 375°F. Coat a sheet pan with cooking spray.

2. In a small skillet, toast the panko over low heat until crispy and browned.

3. Transfer the panko to a shallow bowl and stir in ½ teaspoon of salt. Crack the eggs into a second shallow bowl and whisk together. Spread the almond flour in a third bowl. Set up an assembly line for dredging the pork.

4. Take each piece of pork and dip first in the almond flour, followed by the egg, and then the panko. Set on the greased sheet pan as you work.

5. Transfer to the oven and bake until the coating is golden and the pork is cooked but still juicy, about 10 minutes (depending on the thickness of the pork).

6. Meanwhile, in a bowl, toss together the arugula and tomatoes. In a small bowl, whisk together the oil, vinegar, and remaining ½ teaspoon of salt. Drizzle the dressing over the greens.

7. Once the meat is cooked, let it rest for 5 minutes before slicing and serve atop the salad. Add a squeeze of lemon juice, if desired.

Ingredient tip: Very thin, cutlet-style boneless pork chops work best here. If you can only find the thicker boneless chops, consider slicing or pounding them thinner before coating.

Per Serving: Calories: 634; Fat: 36g; Saturated Fat: 7.5g; Cholesterol: 190mg; Carbohydrates: 23g; Fiber: 3.5g; Protein: 53g; Sodium: 785mg

Beef and Broccoli Stir-Fry

Fast, Nut-Free

Craving Chinese takeout? No need! Try this take on the classic beef and broccoli. The bulk of the ingredients below make up the sauce you'll use to sauté the beef and broccoli, so don't get overwhelmed when peeking at the list. It will come together fast and be packed with flavor.

SERVES 4   *Prep time: 10 minutes / Cook time: 15 minutes*

¼ cup tamari

¼ cup coconut aminos

4 tablespoons freshly squeezed lime juice

2 tablespoons sesame oil

4 garlic cloves, put through a press

2 teaspoons ground ginger (or a 2-inch fresh ginger, grated or minced)

1 teaspoon red pepper flakes (optional)

2 tablespoons coconut oil

2 pounds flank steak, thinly sliced against the grain

½ teaspoon sea salt

½ teaspoon freshly ground black pepper

8 cups chopped broccoli

1. In a bowl, whisk together the tamari, coconut aminos, lime juice, sesame oil, garlic, ginger, and red pepper flakes (if using). Set aside.

2. In a large skillet, heat the coconut oil over medium heat. Season the beef with salt and black pepper. Once the oil is shimmering, add the beef and quickly sear, less than 1 minute per side. (Do not overcrowd the meat; you may need to do this in batches.) Once seared, remove from the pan and set aside.

3. Leave the beef juices in the pan, and add the broccoli and half of the tamari sauce. Cover and simmer until the vegetables start to soften, about 5 minutes.

4. Add the remaining sauce and return the beef to the pan. Bring everything to a boil to thicken the sauce, then remove from the heat. Serve hot.

Ingredient tip: Don't be shy to ask the butcher to slice your beef for you, or look for presliced beef—it makes the cooking go even faster.

Variation tip: Don't feel limited to broccoli. I'll often make this using a prechopped bag of stir-fry vegetables and add some extra broccoli to the mix to bulk it up.

Per Serving: Calories: 516; Fat: 32g; Saturated Fat: 14g; Cholesterol: 96mg; Carbohydrates: 13g; Fiber: 3.5g; Protein: 44g; Sodium: 1,703mg

Slow-Roasted Lamb and Green Beans

Nut-Free

Don't overlook the benefits (and deliciousness) of lamb. While it certainly is an excellent source of protein, it also contains a variety of vitamins, and even a surprising amount of omega-3 fats. This dish is fairly hands-off, but the key is to not rush the process. This is the perfect meal to cook on a cozy weekend at home, not when you're rushing home late and tired from work.

SERVES 4 *Prep time: 15 minutes / Cook time: 1 hour*

2 tablespoons extra-virgin olive oil

1 large onion, sliced

1 teaspoon sea salt

2 pounds boneless lamb shoulder (see Tip)

1 (8-ounce) can tomato sauce

1 (15-ounce) can crushed tomatoes

1½ pounds green beans

1 pound small red potatoes, quartered

1 teaspoon chopped fresh mint

1 teaspoon chopped fresh parsley

Dairy-Free Tzatziki (optional; page 133)

1. In a large Dutch oven, heat the oil over medium heat. Add the onion, salt, and lamb to sear the outside.

2. Add the tomato sauce and crushed tomatoes so they are surrounding the lamb. Bring to a boil and then reduce to a simmer, until the meat starts to become tender, about 30 minutes.

3. Add the green beans and potatoes. Return to a boil, then reduce again to a simmer, cover, and cook until the meat is very tender and has an internal temperature of 160°F, about 30 minutes.

4. Remove from the heat and sprinkle with fresh mint and parsley. If desired, serve with a dollop of tzatziki.

Ingredient tip: Ask your butcher to slice a whole lamb shoulder into four pieces about 8 ounces each for faster cooking and easier serving.

Per Serving: Calories: 560; Fat: 23g; Saturated Fat: 7.5g; Cholesterol: 122mg; Carbohydrates: 45g; Fiber: 11g; Protein: 45g; Sodium: 1,300mg

Basics

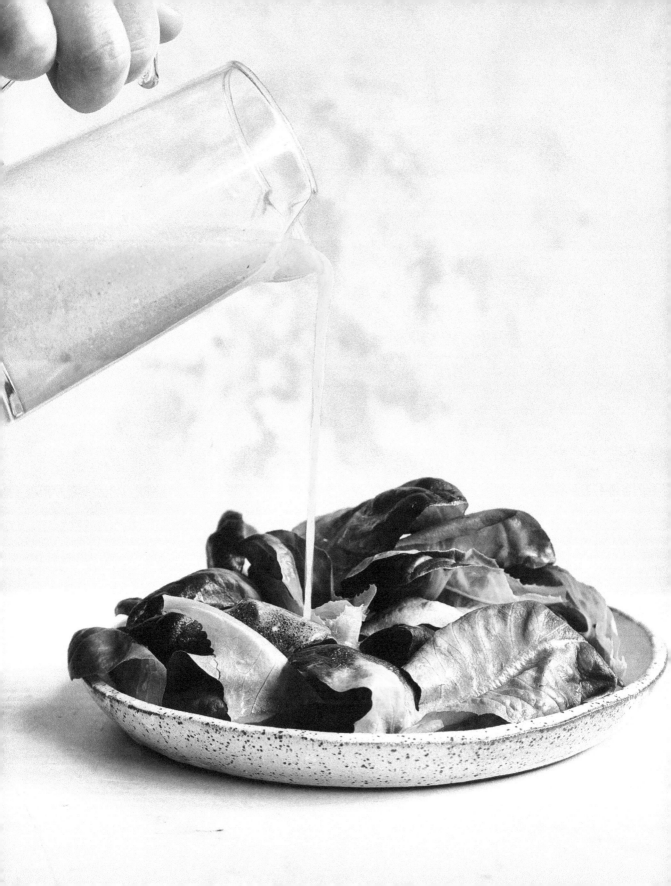

Champagne Vinaigrette

Fast, Vegan, Nut-Free

This is my go-to salad dressing. I whip up several batches weekly and it goes on 90 percent of the quick salads I throw together. While apple cider or balsamic are more common, I love champagne for its light flavor. It's not overbearing and pairs so nicely with a robust olive oil and a touch of sweetness from a natural sweetener. And, this dressing is better for you than nearly any store-bought dressing, which typically are made with refined sugars, unhealthy oils, and unnecessary artificial preservatives.

MAKES ⅔ CUP   *Prep time: 5 minutes*

¼ cup Champagne vinegar

¼ cup extra-virgin olive oil

2 tablespoons water

1 tablespoon Dijon mustard

2 teaspoons honey or maple syrup

1 teaspoon sea salt

½ teaspoon freshly ground black pepper

In a screw-top jar, combine the vinegar, oil, water, mustard, honey, salt, and pepper. Shake well to combine. Use immediately or refrigerate for up to 1 week.

Ingredient tip: When buying honey, choose organic, because it's the only guarantee you're getting pure honey with no undesirable added ingredients. Avoid any "honey" that adds corn, rice, high fructose corn syrup, or any other type of sugar.

Variation tip: Try swapping in balsamic or apple cider vinegar for champagne vinegar. Use what you have on hand and get creative.

Per Serving (2 tablespoons): Calories: 111; Fat: 11g; Saturated Fat: 1.5g; Cholesterol: 0mg; Carbohydrates: 3g; Fiber: 0g; Protein: 0g; Sodium: 538mg

Creamy Lemon-Tahini Dressing

Fast, Vegan, Nut-Free

Tahini is a seed butter that you'll often find in the peanut butter aisle. It's made from sesame seeds, rich in flavor, and pairs well with both sweet and savory dishes. Beyond being scrumptious, it also offers some great nutritional boosts to your body; for instance, it's high in antioxidants, which help your heart and fight inflammation. Drizzle this dressing on roasted veggies, cold salads, meats, and tofu. Add the ginger for a spicy variation.

MAKES ½ CUP   *Prep time: 5 minutes*

3 tablespoons tahini, at room temperature

1 tablespoon extra-virgin olive oil

2 tablespoons freshly squeezed lemon juice

2 to 4 tablespoons warm water

1 tablespoon tamari

1 garlic clove, put through a press

1 teaspoon ground ginger or a 1-inch piece of fresh ginger, grated (optional)

In a medium bowl, whisk together the tahini, oil, lemon juice, water, tamari, garlic, and ginger (if using). Pour into a small Mason jar and keep refrigerated until use.

Cooking tip: Using warm water and room temperature tahini makes this much easier. If you are going for a thicker dip or dressing, add less water. More water will yield a thinner, dressing-like consistency.

Per Serving (2 tablespoons): Calories: 102; Fat: 9g; Saturated Fat: 1.5g; Cholesterol: 0mg; Carbohydrates: 3g; Fiber: 0.5g; Protein: 2g; Sodium: 256mg

Dairy-Free Tzatziki

Fast, Vegan, Nut-Free

Fresh herbs bring any meal to life, especially dill. This is a dairy-free spin on the classic Greek sauce, combining cucumber, dill, and lemon. Here, I recommend using a nondairy yogurt, but if and when you reintroduce dairy back into your diet, feel free to use a plain nonfat yogurt in its place.

MAKES ABOUT 1½ CUPS   *Prep time: 10 minutes*

⅔ cup plain
nondairy yogurt

3 tablespoons avocado
oil mayonnaise

1 tablespoon extra-virgin
olive oil

1 tablespoon freshly
squeezed lemon juice

½ cup fresh dill, minced

½ cup shredded or grated
cucumber

1 garlic clove, put through
a press or minced

1 teaspoon sea salt

½ teaspoon freshly ground
black pepper

In a bowl, stir together the yogurt, mayonnaise, oil, lemon juice, dill, cucumber, garlic, salt, and pepper. Serve or refrigerate for later use. Tzatziki will keep in the refrigerator for 3 to 4 days.

Ingredient tip: There are lots of mayonnaise options on the shelf today. I prefer a mayonnaise containing nothing artificial and made from non-GMO (genetically modified) ingredients, and one that uses avocado oil in place of canola or soy oils.

Per Serving (2 tablespoons): Calories: 41; Fat: 4.5g; Saturated Fat: 0.5g; Cholesterol: 4mg; Carbohydrates: 1g; Fiber: 0.5g; Protein: 0g; Sodium: 217mg

Any Meat Marinade

Fast, Nut-Free

It's well worth the 5 minutes it takes to make this marinade. It both tenderizes your meat and infuses it with incredible flavor. For no cleanup fuss, you can make the marinade right in a resealable plastic bag, add the meat to the bag, and let it marinate in the refrigerator for 2 to 4 hours. No worries if you didn't plan ahead; even just 10 to 20 minutes of sitting in this sauce makes a difference. This recipe makes enough to marinate 2 to 4 pounds of meat.

MAKES ABOUT ¾ CUP   *Prep time: 5 minutes*

¼ cup Worcestershire sauce

¼ cup extra-virgin olive oil

2 tablespoons tamari

2 tablespoons balsamic vinegar

1 tablespoon Dijon mustard

1 or 2 garlic cloves, minced

½ teaspoon sea salt

½ teaspoon freshly ground black pepper

1. In a resealable plastic bag or whatever you're using to marinate your meat, combine the Worcestershire sauce, oil, tamari, vinegar, mustard, garlic, salt, and pepper.

2. Add the meat and marinate for at least 20 minutes (but ideally 2 to 4 hours) in the refrigerator.

Per Serving (1 tablespoon): Calories: 50; Fat: 4.5g; Saturated Fat: 0.5g; Cholesterol: 0mg; Carbohydrates: 2g; Fiber: 0g; Protein: 0g; Sodium: 351mg

Everyday Pasta Sauce

Vegan, Nut-Free

People are often shocked when I tell them that many store-bought pasta and pizza sauces are loaded with added (and unnecessary) sugars. This is such a basic recipe and one of my top nutrition-improving tips, so double the batch if you can. Divide it into freezer-safe containers and you'll be stocked for a month.

MAKES ABOUT 5 CUPS   *Prep time: 5 minutes / Cook time: 30 minutes*

3 tablespoons extra-virgin olive oil

3 garlic cloves, put through a press or minced

1 teaspoon sea salt

1 (28–ounce) can crushed tomatoes

1 cup water

2 large fresh basil leaves

1. In a large pot, heat the oil over medium-low heat. Add the garlic and salt, and sauté the garlic for 1 to 2 minutes until fragrant (garlic can easily burn, so keep the heat low).

2. Add the tomatoes and stir briefly to absorb the flavors. Then, add the water and basil leaves. Increase the heat to high and bring to a boil. Reduce the heat to low and let simmer uncovered for 30 minutes to thicken the sauce. Add additional salt to taste, if needed.

Storage tip: This sauce will freeze well. Let cool completely before transferring to freezer-safe containers. Label the date you made it and store for up to 3 months.

Per Serving (1 cup): Calories: 133; Fat: 8g; Saturated Fat: 1g; Cholesterol: 0mg; Carbohydrates: 12g; Fiber: 4g; Protein: 3g; Sodium: 767mg

Peanut Sauce

Fast, Vegan

This sauce enhances simple roasted tofu, chicken, or veggies. And the recipe is versatile. I love swapping tamari for coconut aminos (which offers a slightly sweeter flavor), or almond butter for the peanut butter. You'll also see that I've included some optional ingredients that can add depth to the flavor.

MAKES ABOUT ½ CUP   *Prep time: 5 minutes*

¼ cup peanut butter, preferably natural

2 tablespoons tamari

2 to 3 tablespoons warm water (less for thicker sauce)

1 tablespoon freshly squeezed lime juice

1 teaspoon honey

1 teaspoon sesame oil (optional)

1 teaspoon sriracha (optional), for seasoning

In a medium bowl, whisk together the peanut butter, tamari, water, lime juice, honey, sesame oil (if using), and sriracha (if using). Pour into a small Mason jar and keep refrigerated until use, up to 1 week.

Ingredient tip: Tamari is gluten-free soy sauce. You'll find it in the same grocery aisle as soy sauce and it tastes identical. Of course, check the label to make sure it is gluten-free, as some brands are not.

Per Serving (1 tablespoon): Calories: 58; Fat: 4g; Saturated Fat: 0.5g; Cholesterol: 0mg; Carbohydrates: 2g; Fiber: 0.5g; Protein: 2g; Sodium: 278mg

Spinach-Walnut Pesto

Fast, Vegan

A healthier spin on classic pesto, this sauce uses baby spinach and replaces pine nuts with walnuts. You can leave out the basil and increase the amount of baby spinach by 1 cup, though I love the taste of basil in it. You'll notice that there's no cheese in here, to keep it dairy-free, but my guess is you won't even miss it.

MAKES ABOUT 1 CUP   *Prep time: 10 minutes*

⅓ cup walnuts, toasted (see Tip)

1 cup tightly packed fresh basil leaves

3 cups baby spinach

2 garlic cloves, peeled but whole

2 tablespoons freshly squeezed lemon juice

1 teaspoon sea salt

2 tablespoons extra-virgin olive oil

2 to 4 tablespoons water

1. In a food processor or blender, combine the walnuts, basil, spinach, garlic, lemon juice, and salt and blend until the ingredients come together. Scrape down the sides of the blender and with the machine running, slowly add the oil, followed by 2 tablespoons of water and process until blended.

2. If your sauce still seems very thick, add an additional 1 to 2 tablespoons of water until you reach your desired consistency.

Ingredient tip: Toasted nuts taste far better than raw, and it's well worth the extra time. You can toast the walnuts either in the oven at 350°F or in a skillet over medium-low heat. Toasting will take anywhere from 5 to 10 minutes. Stir them once or twice, and watch them carefully as they can burn quickly. Use right away or store in an airtight container for up to 3 days; they'll last even longer in the freezer.

Storage tip: You can divide leftover pesto into ice cube trays. On nights when you need a fast meal, thaw 2 or 3 cubes and toss into your favorite plate of roasted vegetables, over pasta, or even use it to marinate meat. The possibilities are endless.

Per Serving (2 tablespoons): Calories: 64; Fat: 6g; Saturated Fat: 0.5g; Cholesterol: 0mg; Carbohydrates: 2g; Fiber: 1g; Protein: 1g; Sodium: 307mg

Easy Roasted Spaghetti Squash

Vegan, Nut-Free

This is a plan-ahead recipe because it takes 1 hour to bake. But once it's cooked, you can pull together quick and easy weeknight meals in no time. Spaghetti squash is low in calories and has a fairly neutral flavor, which makes it a great base for any sauce you love. Top it with a red sauce and Garlicky Green Turkey Meatballs (page 97), a flavor-forward Spinach-Walnut Pesto (page 137), or salsa, guacamole, and Salsa Verde Shredded Pork (page 117).

SERVES 4   *Prep time: 5 minutes / Cook time: 1 hour*

1 large spaghetti squash

½ cup water

2 tablespoons extra-virgin olive oil

1 teaspoon sea salt

1 teaspoon freshly ground black pepper

1. Preheat the oven to 350°F.

2. Very carefully halve the squash lengthwise, and use a fork to loosen and discard the strings and seeds. Pour the water in the bottom of a baking pan and place the squash facedown.

3. Bake for 1 hour (the skin will slightly brown and feel soft to the touch).

4. Let the squash cool. Once cooled, flip the squash and use a fork to scrape out the flesh (it will look like spaghetti strands) into a large bowl.

5. Toss the strands with oil, salt, and pepper.

6. Serve immediately or, once cooled, place in an air-tight container in the refrigerator. It will keep for up to 5 days.

Per Serving: Calories: 184; Fat: 9g; Saturated Fat: 1.5g; Cholesterol: 0mg; Carbohydrates: 28g; Fiber: 6g; Protein: 3g; Sodium: 650mg

Coconut Cauliflower Rice

Fast, Vegan, Nut-Free

While it's definitely not rice, riced cauliflower makes a really nice low-carb alternative for dishes that are typically rice-based. The coconut milk here makes the dish creamy and will keep you full and satisfied. This dish pairs superbly with Weeknight Salmon Stir-Fry (page 89) and Coconut Thai Curry Mussels (page 93).

SERVES 2   *Prep time: 5 minutes / Cook time: 15 to 20 minutes*

1 tablespoon coconut oil

1 (10-ounce) bag frozen riced cauliflower

½ teaspoon sea salt, plus more as needed

⅓ cup canned full-fat coconut milk

¼ teaspoon freshly ground black pepper, plus more as needed

1. In a medium saucepan, heat the oil over medium heat. Add the frozen cauliflower and salt and sauté on medium-low heat until the cauliflower becomes tender, about 10 minutes.

2. Add the coconut milk and reduce the heat to a low simmer. Continue to stir occasionally until the cauliflower starts to absorb some of the milk and the liquid reduces, about 5 minutes longer.

3. Season with the pepper and more salt, if desired, and serve.

Variation tip: You can skip the coconut milk and just sauté the riced cauliflower in oil, salt, and pepper over medium-low heat until it gets tender, and serve.

Per Serving: Calories: 179; Fat: 15g; Saturated Fat: 13g; Cholesterol: 0mg; Carbohydrates: 9g; Fiber: 3g; Protein: 3g; Sodium: 635mg

Crispy Tofu

Fast, Vegan, Nut-Free

Tofu is a great way to add protein and staying power to any meal. This versatile recipe is found in Greek Goulash with Crispy Baked Tofu (page 83) and Buddha Bowls (page 85). I also often like to keep a batch prepared in the refrigerator to add to quick weeknight meals or as a salad topping for an easy lunch.

SERVES 4 *Prep time: 5 minutes / Cook time: 15 minutes*

1 (14-ounce) block extra-firm tofu

1 tablespoon extra-virgin olive oil

½ teaspoon sea salt

1. Drain the water from the package of tofu. Wrap the block in a clean kitchen towel and gently press down to remove some of the excess water.

2. Remove the towel and slice the block into cubes (any size you want; though the smaller you make them, the crispier they become).

3. In a large skillet (either nonstick or seasoned cast iron), heat the oil over medium heat. Add the tofu and sprinkle with the salt. Let the tofu cook without moving for 3 to 4 minutes.

4. Checking to make sure the skillet-side down pieces are lightly browned, flip the tofu to the next side and continue the process until all the sides are browned and getting crispy. The entire process should take 10 to 15 minutes, depending on the size of your tofu cubes.

5. Serve immediately or let cool completely before refrigerating.

Ingredient tip: For extra crispy tofu, try pressing your tofu under some weight for 1 to 2 hours. I like to place wrapped tofu under a cutting board (for even pressure) and then place some heavier pots or pans on top.

Per Serving: Calories: 127; Fat: 8.5g; Saturated Fat: 1g; Cholesterol: 0mg; Carbohydrates: 2g; Fiber: 1g; Protein: 10g; Sodium: 295mg

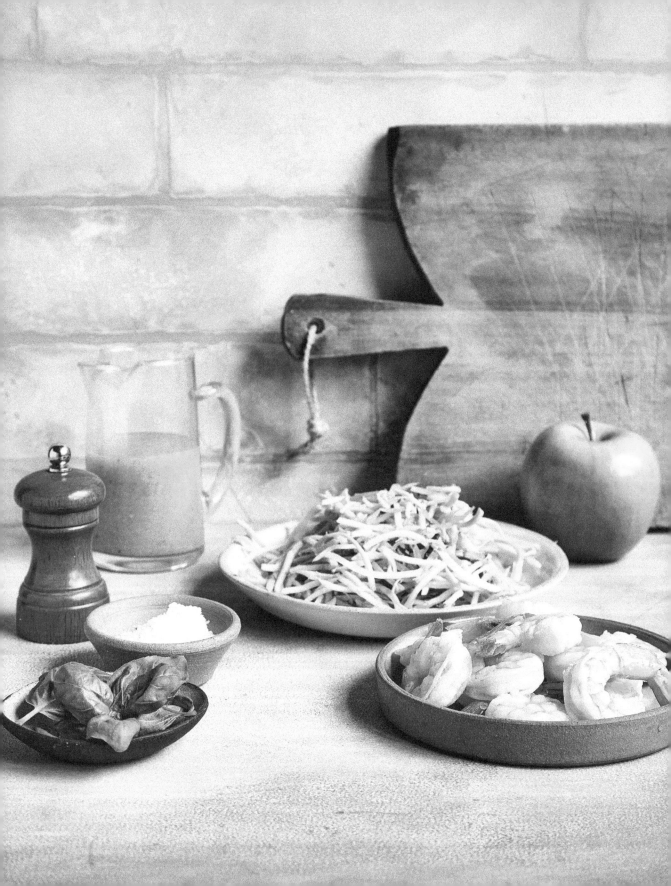

Measurement Conversions

VOLUME EQUIVALENTS (LIQUID)

US Standard (ounces)	US Standard (approximate)	Metric
2 tablespoons	1 fl.oz.	30 mL
¼ cup	2 fl. oz.	60 mL
½ cup	4 fl. oz.	120 mL
1 cup	8 fl. oz.	240 mL
1½ cups	12 fl.oz.	355 mL
2 cups or 1 pint	16 fl. oz.	475 mL
4 cups or 1 quart	32 fl. oz.	1 L
1 gallon	128 fl.oz.	4 L

OVEN TEMPERATURES

Fahrenheit (F)	Celsius (C) (approximate)
250°F	120°C
300°F	150°C
325°F	165°C
350°F	180°C
375°F	190°C
400°F	200°C
425°F	220°C
450°F	230°C

VOLUME EQUIVALENTS (DRY)

US Standard	Metric (approximate)
⅛ teaspoon	0.5 mL
¼ teaspoon	1 mL
½ teaspoon	2 mL
¾ teaspoon	4 mL
1 teaspoon	5 mL
1 tablespoon	15 mL
¼ cup	60 mL
⅓ cup	79 mL
½ cup	120 mL
⅔ cup	156 mL
¾ cup	177 mL
1 cup	240 mL
2 cups or 1 pint	475 mL
3 cups	700 mL
4 cups or 1 quart	1 L

WEIGHT EQUIVALENTS

US Standard	Metric (approximate)
½ ounce	15 g
1 ounce	30 g
2 ounces	60 g
4 ounces	115 g
8 ounces	225 g
12 ounces	340 g
16 ounces or 1 pound	455 g

References

Augustin L. S. A., et al. "Glycemic Index, Glycemic Load and Glycemic Response: An International Scientific Consensus Summit from the International Carbohydrate Quality Consortium (ICQC)." *Nutrition, Metabolism & Cardiovascular Diseases* 25, no. 9 (September 2015): 795-815. doi: 10.1016/j.numecd.2015.05.005.

Barbaro, Maria Raffaella, et al. "Recent Advances in Understanding Non-Celiac Gluten Sensitivity." *F1000Research* 11, no. 7 (October 2018): 1631. doi: 10.12688/f1000research.15849.1.

Bordoni, Alessandra, Francesca Danesi, Dominique Dardevet, Didier Dupont, Aida Fernandez, Doreen Gille, Claudia Nunes Dos Santos, Paula Pinto, Roberta Re, Didier Rémond, et. al. "Dairy Products and Inflammation: A Review of the Clinical Evidence." *Critical Reviews in Food Science and Nutrition* 57, no. 12 (August 2015): 2497-2525. doi: 10.1080/10408398.2014.967385.

Caballero, Benjamin, Paul Finglas, and Fidel Toldra. *Encyclopedia of Food and Health*. Waltham, MA: Academic Press, 2015.

"Essential Fatty Acids." lpi.oregonstate.edu/mic/other-nutrients/essential-fatty-acids.

Foodsafety.gov. "Safe Minimum Cooking Temperature Charts." Foodsafety.gov/food-safety-charts/safe-minimum-cooking-temperature.

Foodsafety.gov. "Keep Food Safe." Foodsafety.gov/keep-food-safe.

Givens, D. Ian, et al. *Health Benefits of Organic Food: Effects of the Environment*. Oxford: CAB International, 2008.

Harvard Health Publishing. "Should You Go Organic?" Published September 2015. Health.Harvard.edu/staying-healthy/should-you-go-organic.

Health.com. "The Burning Question: Do I Need to Buy Organic Chicken?" Published April 27, 2011. Health.com/nutrition/the-burning-question-do-i-need-to-buy-organic-chicken.

Jenkins, D. J. A., et al. "The Relation of Low Glycaemic Index Fruit Consumption to Glycaemic Control and Risk Factors for Coronary Heart Disease in type 2 Diabetes." *Diabetologia* 54 (2011): 271-279. doi: 10.1007/s00125-010-1927-1.

Karl, J. Philip, and Edward Saltzman. "The Role of Whole Grains in Body Weight Regulation." *Advances in Nutrition* 3, no. 5 (September 2012): 697-707. doi: 10.3945/an.112.002782.

Leheska, J. M., L. D. Thompson, J. C. Howe, E. Hentges, J. Boyce, J. C. Brooks, B. Shriver, L. Hoover, and M. F. Miller. "Effects of Conventional and Grass-Feeding Systems on the Nutrient Composition of Beef." *Journal of Animal Science* 86, no. 12 (December 2008): 3575-3585. doi: 10.2527/jas.2007-0565.

Li, Thomas S.C. *Vegetables and Fruits: Nutritional and Therapeutic Values.* Boca Raton, FL: CRC Press, 2008.

National Center for Complementary and Integrative Health. "NIH Fact Sheet—Soy." nccih.nih.gov/health/soy/ataglance.htm

National Institutes of Health. "NIH Fact Sheet—Omega-3 Fatty Acids." ods.od.nih.gov/factsheets/Omega3FattyAcids-HealthProfessional.

The Nutrition Source (blog). "Coffee." Harvard T.H. Chan School of Public Health. hsph.harvard.edu/nutritionsource/food-features/coffee.

Poti, Jennifer M., et al. "Ultra-Processed Food Intake and Obesity: What Really Matters for Health-Processing or Nutrient Content?" *Current Obesity Reports* 6, no. 4 (December 2017): 420–431. doi: 10.1007/s13679-017-0285-4.

Réhault-Godbert, Sophie, Nicolas Guyot, and Yves Nys. "The Golden Egg: Nutritional Value, Bioactivities, and Emerging Benefits for Human Health." *Nutrients* 11, no. 3 (March 22, 2019): 684. doi: 10.3390/nu11030684.

Rippe, James M., and Theodore J. Angelopoulos. "Relationship between Added Sugars Consumption and Chronic Disease Risk Factors: Current Understanding." *Nutrients* 8, no. 11 (November 2016): 697. doi: 10.3390/nu8110697.

Rolfes, Sharon Rady, Kathryn Pinna, and Eleanor Noss Whitney. *Understanding Normal and Clinical Nutrition*, 9th ed. Belmont, CA: Wadsworth, Cengage Learning, 2012.

Shan Z., C. D. Rehm, G. Rogers, M. Ruan, D. D. Wang, F. B. Hu, D. Mozaffarian, F. F. Zhang, and S. N. Bhupathiraju. "Trends in Dietary Carbohydrate, Protein, and Fat Intake and Diet Quality Among US Adults, 1999–2016." *JAMA* 322, no. 12 (August 31, 2019): 1178–1187. doi: 10.1001/jama.2019.13771.

Stanhope, Kimber L. "Sugar Consumption, Metabolic Disease and Obesity: The State of the Controversy." *Critical Reviews in Clinical Laboratory Sciences* 53, no. 1 (February 2016): 52-67. doi: 10.3109/10408363.2015.1084990.

Thornton, Simon N. "Increased Hydration Can Be Associated with Weight Loss." *Frontiers in Nutrition* 10, no. 3 (June 10, 2016): 18. doi: 10.3389/fnut.2016.00018.

USDA Food Safety and Inspection Service. "USDA Food Temperature Reference." fsis.usda.gov/wps/portal/fsis/topics/food-safety-education/get-answers/food-safety -fact-sheets/safe-food-handling/safe-minimum-internal-temperature-chart /ct_index.

Vaclavik, Vickie A., Marjorie M. Devine, and Marcia H. Pimentel. *Dimensions of Food,* 5th ed. Boca Raton, FL: CRC Press, 2002.

Index

Acknowledgments

Pursuing my passion for nutrition is what got me to this point today, authoring a book, and none of it would have been possible without the experiences that have led me here. To my husband, John, who encouraged me to follow my dream and go back to school. To the University of Michigan School of Public Health, which educated me into becoming an expert in this field. To my past and current employers who shaped my skills, and to every individual I've ever worked with through my personal private practice. Everyone who has touched me at all those points in some way educated me, guided me, and carried me to where I am today. I am forever grateful.

About the Author

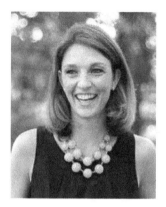

Kim McDevitt is a registered dietitian with a passion for guiding people on how to more easily make cleaner, better-for-you wellness choices. She brings a full range of experience and insight to her work as a registered dietitian, nutrition coach, and educator, both in private practice and with brands.

She has over seven years of experience working on nutrition strategy and education, content development, and consumer and media relations, supporting the initiatives of many brands. Her insights as a nutrition expert and consumer advocate add value to all of her work, and she's a passionate advocate for clean labels and healthier products. When she's not scrutinizing labels or sussing out the latest clean-label products, Kim spends time running, skiing, cooking, and chasing after her three young kids. She calls Portland, Maine, home and has no plans for leaving anytime soon.

CPSIA information can be obtained
at www.ICGtesting.com
Printed in the USA
JSHW041750110820
7185JS00003B/11